LAST WATCH
OF THE NIGHT

ALSO BY PAUL MONETTE

POEMS

The Carpenter at the Asylum
No Witnesses
Love Alone: 18 Elegies for Rog

NOVELS

Taking Care of Mrs. Carroll
The Gold Diggers
The Long Shot
Lightfall
Afterlife
Halfway Home

NONFICTION

Borrowed Time: An AIDS Memoir
Becoming a Man: Half a Life Story

LAST WATCH OF THE NIGHT

Essays Too Personal and Otherwise

PAUL MONETTE

A Harvest Book
Harcourt Brace & Company
San Diego   New York   London

The book's epigraph, from *Collected Poems* by Frank O'Hara, copyright © 1971 by Maureen Granville-Smith, Administratrix of the Estate of Frank O'Hara, is reprinted by permission of Alfred A. Knopf, Inc. The quotes from Sappho are from Mary Barnard, *Sappho: A New Translation;* copyright © 1958 The Regents of the University of California; © renewed 1984 Mary Barnard; reprinted by permission of the Regents of the University of California and the University of California Press. The quote from "The Road Not Taken" is from *The Poetry of Robert Frost,* edited by Edward Connery Lathem; copyright 1944 by Robert Frost; copyright 1916, 1969 by Henry Holt and Company, Inc.; reprinted by permission of Henry Holt and Company, Inc. The quote from *Private Lives* copyright © 1930 by Noel Coward is reprinted by permission of Michael Imison Playwrights Ltd., 28 Almeida Street, London N1 1TD. The quotes from "Ithaka" are from C.P. Cavafy, *Collected Poems,* translated by Edmund Keeley and Philip Sherrard; copyright © 1975 by Keeley/Sherrard, revised edn. 1992; reprinted by permission of Princeton University Press. The lines from "Deer Lay Down Their Bones" are from *Selected Poems* by Robinson Jeffers; copyright © 1954 by Robinson Jeffers; reprinted by permission of Random House, Inc. The last two stanzas of "Moriturus" by Edna St. Vincent Millay are from *Collected Poems,* Harper & Row; copyright © 1928, 1955 by Edna St. Vincent Millay and Norma Millay Ellis; reprinted by permission of Elizabeth Barnett, literary executor. The quote from Fran Lebowitz is used with her permission.

Library of Congress Cataloging-in-Publication Data
Monette, Paul.
Last watch of the night: essays / by Paul Monette. — 1st ed.
p. cm.
ISBN 0-15-600202-7
I. Title
PS3563.O523L3   1994
814´.54—dc20   93-47655

Designed by Lydia D'moch
Printed in the United States of America
First Harvest edition 1995
A B C D E

Once again for Winston

keeper of myth
who had a great idea

CONTENTS

ACKNOWLEDGMENTS

The author wishes to express his gratitude for the good graces of several people who gave invaluable support and inspiration to the writing of this book. *Frontiers* (and especially its editor, David Kalmansohn), where "Puck" first appeared. Merloyd Lawrence, for generously sharing her memories of Aunt Gert. Tad Mosel, for his definitive life of Katharine Cornell—*Leading Lady* (Atlantic–Little Brown, 1978)—written with Gertrude Macy. Brother Toby, Sister Marti, and Sister Julie, whose mission at Starcross Community is a wonder of light out of darkness. Bishop Otis Charles, for his great personal courage in single-handedly changing the balance in the House of Bishops. Ma Jaya and her tireless workers at Kashi Ranch, for the blessings they've brought to a suffering people. Neil Baldwin, Executive Director of the National Book Foundation, for uncountable kindnesses and efficiency in shepherding my lecture at the Library of Congress. The Op-Ed staff at *The New York Times*, where a portion of "The Politics of Silence" first appeared. Laurence Goldstein and the staff of the *Michigan Quarterly Review,* where "Mustering" first appeared. My doctors—especially James Thommes, Robert Jenkins, and Aaron Aronow—for keeping my head above water. And Barbara Horwitz, diagnostician *sine qua non.* Tony Johnson, for his gift of humor in calamitous times and the brave example of his own writing. Wendy Weil, my agent and friend for twenty years, for her staunch enthusiasm and her great heart. Finally, Drenka Willen, my editor at Harcourt Brace, for her intellectual rigor and unfailing good humor in the service of keeping me honest.

When I die, don't come, I wouldn't want a leaf
to turn away from the sun—it loves it there.
There's nothing so spiritual about being happy
but you can't miss a day of it, because it doesn't last.

—*Frank O'Hara*

PUCK

STEVIE HAD BEEN in the hospital for about a week and a half, diagnosed with PCP, his first full-blown infection. For some reason he wasn't responding to the standard medication, and his doctors had put him on some new exotic combination regimen—one side effect of which was to turn his piss blue. He certainly didn't act or feel sick, except for a little breathlessness. He was still miles from the brink of death. Not even showing any sign of late-stage shriveling up—let alone the ravages of end-stage, where all that's left of life is sleep shot through with delirium.

Stevie was reading the paper, in a larky mood because he'd just had a dose of Ativan. I was sitting by the window, doodling with a script that I had to finish quickly in order to keep my insurance. "I miss Puck," he announced to no one in particular, no response required.

And I stopped writing and looked out the window at the heat-blistered parking lot, the miasma of low smog bleaching the hills in the distance. "You think Puck's going to survive me?"

"Yup," he replied. Which startled me, a bristle of the old denial that none of us was going to die just yet. Even though we were all living our lives in "dog years" now, seven for every twelvemonth, I still couldn't feel my own death as a palpable thing. To have undertaken the fight as we had for better drugs and treatment, so that we had become a guerrilla tribe of amateur microbiologists, pharmacist/shamans, our own best healers—there were those of us who'd convinced ourselves in 1990 that the dying was soon going to stop.

AIDS, you see, was on the verge of becoming a "chronic manageable illness." That was our totem mantra after we buried the second wave, or was it the third? When I met Steve Kolzak on the Fourth of July in '88, he told me he had seven friends who were going to die in the next six months—and they did. It was my job to persuade him that we could fall in love anyway, embracing between the bombs. And then we would pitch our tent in the chronic, manageable clearing, years and years given back to us by the galloping strides of science. No more afflicted than a diabetic, the daily insulin keeping him one step ahead of his body.

So don't tell me I had less time than a ten-year-old dog— admittedly one who was a specimen of roaring good health, still out chasing coyotes in the canyon every night, his watchman's bark at home sufficient to curdle the blood. But if I was angry at Stevie for saying so, I kept it to myself as the hospital stay dragged on. A week of treatment for PCP became two, and he found himself reaching more and more for the oxygen. Our determination, or mine at least, to see this bout as a minor inconvenience remained unshaken. Stevie upped his Ativan and mostly retained his playful demeanor, though woe to the nurse or technician who thought a stream of happy talk would get them through the holocaust. Stevie's bark was as lethal as Puck's if you said the wrong thing.

And he didn't get better, either, because it wasn't pneumonia that was killing him. I woke up late on Friday, the fifteenth of September, to learn they'd moved him to intensive care, and I raced to the hospital to find him in a panic, fear glazing his flashing Irish eyes as he clutched the oxygen cup to his mouth. They pulled him through the crisis with steroids, but still wouldn't say what the problem was. Some nasty bug that a sewer of antibiotics hadn't completely arrested yet. But surely all it required was a little patience till one of these drugs kicked in.

His family arrived from back East, the two halves of the divorce. Yet it looked as if the emergency had passed, such is the false promise of massive steroids. I mean, he looked *fine*. He was impish and animated all through the weekend; it was we who had to be vigilant lest he get too tired. And I was so manically certain that he'd pull through, I could hardly take it in at first when one of the docs, shifty-eyed, refined the diagnosis: "He's having a toxic reaction to the chemo."

The chemo? But how could that be? They'd been treating his KS for sixteen months, till all the lesions were under control. Even the ones on his face: you had to know they were there to spot them, a scatter of faded purple under his beard. Besides, KS wasn't a sickness really, it was mostly just a nuisance. This was how deeply invested I was in denial, the 1990 edition. Since KS had never landed us in the hospital, it didn't count. And the chemo was the treatment, so how could it be life-threatening?

Easily, as it turned out. The milligram dosage of bleomycin, a biweekly drip in the doctor's office, is cumulative. After a certain point you run the risk of toxicity, your lungs seizing with fibrous tissue—all the resilience gone till you can't even whistle in the dark anymore. You choke to death the way Stevie did, gasping into the oxygen mask, a little less air with every breath.

Still, there were moments of respite, even on that last day. "I'm not dying, am I?" he asked about noon, genuinely astonished. Finally his doctor came in and broke the news: the damage to the lungs was irreversible, and the most we could hope for was two or three weeks. Stevie nodded and pulled off the mask to speak. "Listen, I'm a greedy bastard," he declared wryly. "I'll take what I can get." As I recall, the idea was to send him home in a wheelchair with an oxygen tank.

I cried when the doctor left, trying to tell him how terrible it was, though he knew it better than I. Yet he smiled and put out a hand to comfort me, reassuring me that he felt no panic. He was on so much medication for pain and anxiety that his own dying had become a movie—a sad one to be sure, but the Ativan/Percodan cocktail was keeping the volume down. I kept saying how much I loved him, as if to store the feeling up for the empty days ahead. Was there anything I could do? Anything left unsaid?

He shook his head, that muzzy wistful smile. Then his eyebrows lifted in surprise: "I'm not going to see Puck again." No regret, just amazement. And then it was time to grab the mask once more, the narrowing tunnel of air, the morphine watch. Twelve hours later he was gone, for death was even greedier than he.

And I was a widower twice now. Nothing for it but to stumble through the week that followed, force-fed by all my anguished friends, pulling together a funeral at the Old North Church at Forest Lawn. A funeral whose orations smeared the blame like dogshit on the rotting churches of this dead Republic, the politicians who run the ovens and dance on our graves. In the limo that took us up the hill to the gravesite, Steve's mother Dolores patted my knee and declared with a ribald trace of an Irish brogue: "Thanks for not burning the flag."

We laughed. A mere oversight, I assured her. She knew that Steve and I had spent a fruitless afternoon the previous Fourth of July—our anniversary, as it happened—going from Thrifty to Target trying to find stars-and-stripes to burn at our party. No such luck: all the flags we found were plastic or polyester, the consistency of cheap shower curtains. A perfect symbol, we realized, of the country we had lost during the decade of the calamity.

We buried the urn of his ashes high on a hill just at the rim of the chaparral, at the foot of a California live oak. The long shadow of our grieving circle fell across the hillside grass where I had buried Roger four years before; the shadow fell on my own grave, as a matter of fact, which is just to the left of Roger's, as if I will one day fling an arm about him and cradle us to sleep. After the putrefaction of the flesh, a pair of skeletons tangled together like metaphysical lovers out of Donne. And my other bone-white arm reaching above my skull, clawing the dirt with piano-key fingers, trying to get to Steve's ashes, just out of reach.

But what has it all got to do with the dog, exactly? My friend Victor stayed with me for the first week of Widowhood II. When at last he went off to juggle the shards of his own dwindling immunity, and I woke to a smudged October morning, my first thought wasn't *Oh poor me,* about which I had already written the book, but rather: *Who's going to take care of Puck?* What nudged me perhaps was the beast himself, who sprawled across the middle of the sagging double bed, permitting me a modest curl of space on the far left side.

You must try to appreciate, I never used to be anything like a rapturist about dogs, Puck or any other. My friend César used to say that Puck was the only dog he knew who'd been raised without any sentimentality at all. I was such a manic creature myself during his formative years that it was all he could do to scramble out of my lurching way, and not take it personally when I'd shoo him away for no reason. This was not the same as having trained him. He rather tumbled up, like one of those squalling babies in Dickens, saved in the nick of time from a scald of boiling water by a harried Mrs. Micawber.

And yet when Roger died, and I thought I had died along with him, the only thing that got me out of bed, groggy at sunset, was that Puck still had to be fed. I could see in his limpid, heartstopping eyes that he knew Roger was not coming back; or maybe he had acquired a permanent wince seeing me sob so inconsolably, hour after hour, gallantly putting his chin on the bed with a questioning look, in case I wanted company. I remember asking my brother in Pennsylvania if the dog could be shipped to him when I died, an event that seemed at the time as close as the walls of this room. But I didn't really like to think of Puck snuffling about in the fields of Bucks County, he whose breeding made him thrive in the desert hills of Southern California.

Half Rhodesian ridgeback, half black lab—or half Zimbabwean ridgeback, I ought to say, since one of my earliest encounters with political correctness occurred in Laurel Canyon Park. In the early eighties it was a place where we could run our dogs off lead, one eye peeled for the panel truck of Animal Control. A sixty-dollar ticket if they caught you—or in this case, if they caught Puck, who left the paying of municipal fines in my capable hands.

He was one of a litter of nine, his mother a purebred ridgeback, tawny and noble, her back bisected by the stiff brush of her ridge, which ran from just behind her shoulders and petered out at her rump. A dog bred to hunt lions, we'd heard, especially prized for being able to go long stretches without any water, loping across the veldt. As a sort of modulation of its terrifying bark, a bay of Baskerville proportions, the ridgeback had developed over time a growl as savage as that of the lions it stalked. Try to get near a ridgeback when he's feeding, you'll see what I mean. You feel like one of those helpless children at the zoo, about to lose an arm through a chain-link fence, waving a box of Crackerjacks in the roaring face of the king.

Ah but you see, there were compensating factors on the father's side. For Nellie, fertile mother of Puck and his eight siblings, had gotten it on with a strapping black lab high up in

Benedict Canyon. A lab who was considered most *déclassé,* perhaps a bit of a half-breed himself, so friendly and ebullient that his people were always in peril of being knocked over or slobbered on. Not at all the sort of genes that Nellie's owners were seeking to rarefy even further. We were told all this in a rush by Nellie's starlet mistress, herself the achingly pretty daughter of a wondrously tucked and lifted movie star of the fifties—a pair who looked like sisters if you squinted, beautiful and not much else, the perfect ticket in L.A. to a long and happy journey on the median strip of life.

This was at a Thanksgiving supper in Echo Park—not the year we found the murdered Latino in the driveway as we left, but I think the year after. In any case, Roger and I had been worrying over the issue of a watchdog for some time now, as a security system cheaper by far than the alarm circuits that wired the hills around us, shrieking falsely into the night. The starlet daughter assured us that ridgebacks were brilliant sentries, ferociously protective.

We went back and forth in the next few weeks, warned by both our families that it was just another thing to tie us down. Besides, we traveled too much, and it wasn't fair to an animal to be getting boarded all the time. None of them understood how stirred we'd been the previous spring, when a whimper brought us to the front door one stormy night. A bedraggled one-eyed Pekingese dripped on the tile, matted and scrawny and quaking in the rain. The most improbable creature, the very last dog that either of us would have chosen. But we couldn't send him back out in the whirlwind either, a bare *hors d'oeuvre* for the sleek coyotes that roamed our canyon in pairs.

We put signs on the trees up and down Kings Road, FOUND instead of the usual LOST (for cats, especially, disappeared with alarming frequency in the hills). Nobody called to claim the one-eyed runt, and it started to look as if we were stuck with him. Without consultation, Roger began to call him Pepper and comb him out. I resisted mightily: *This was not by a long shot what anyone would call a watchdog.* I felt faintly ridiculous walking Pepper with his string leash, as if I'd become an aging queen before my time. Thus I withheld my sentiments rigorously, leaving most of the care and feeding to Roger—though now and again I'd permit the orphan to perch on my lap while I typed.

And then about three weeks later we were strolling up Harold Way, Roger and Pepper and I, past the gates to Liberace's spread. We turned to a cry of delight, as a young black woman came running down the driveway. "Thass my mama dog!" she squealed, scooping the one-eyed dustmop into her arms. In truth, Pepper seemed as overjoyed as she, licking her with abandon. The young woman called uphill to the kitchen yard, summoning her mother: "Grits home!" And a moment later an equally joyous woman came trundling toward us, crisp white uniform and billowing apron worthy of Tara.

No, no, of course we wouldn't dream of taking money. This joyous reunion was all the reward we needed. And so we trudged on home, trying not to feel even more ridiculous as we hastily put away the doll-size bowls by the kitchen door that had held Pepper/Grits's food and water. We laughed it off, or tried to anyway, gushing appropriately when the daughter appeared at our door that evening, bearing a peach pie almost too pretty to eat. "This is like Faulkner," Roger declared as we sliced the bounty. Faulkner, I replied, would not have used a Pekingese.

We never saw Pepper again—never even had the chance to ask how he'd lost that eye. But it goes to show how primed we were at the end of the year, when the starlet called nearly every day to say the litter was going fast. We thought we'd go over and have a look, but the only time the lot of us were free was Christmas morning. "Now we don't have to take one," I admonished Roger as we turned up the dirt road. A minute later we were in the kitchen, inundated by the scrambling of nine puppies. "Pick a lively one," I said, though the sheer explosion of canine anarchy didn't seem to have produced a sluggard or a runt. They squirmed out of our hands and yapped and chased. We couldn't have been said to have actually made a choice. The starlet and her human pups were waiting impatiently in the living room to open their gifts. Roger and I exchanged a shrug, and I reached for the one that was trying to crawl behind the refrigerator.

"You don't owe me anything," the starlet trilled. "Just the fifty bucks for his shots." We waved and promised to send a check, clamoring into the car with our erupting bundle. A black lab followed us barking down the drive. The father, we supposed. "He's not going to be *that* big, is he?" murmured Roger in some dismay. By the time we got home we were calling him Puck, in part because some friends of ours had just named a daughter Ariel, and we'd liked the Shakespearean spin of that, the sense that we were bringing home a changeling. The first thing Puck did when he tottered into the house was make for the Christmas tree, where he squatted and peed on a package from Gump's.

I don't remember a whole lot after that, not for the first five years, so assiduously was I trying to avoid the doggy sort of bathos. I do recall how fretful Roger was for the first six months, waiting for Puck to lift his leg instead of squatting. And the moment of triumph when he finally did, on a bush of wild anis. His main lair was beneath my butcher-block desk in the study—where he lies even as I write this, his head propped uncomfortably on the wooden crossbeam that holds the legs in place. We quickly learned that he wouldn't be budged from any of his makeshift doghouses, which came to include the undercave of every table in the house. A lion's growl of warning if you got too close.

I fed him, I walked him. As I say, I was crazed in those years like a starlet myself, frantic to have a script made, fawning as indiscriminately as a puppy over every self-styled producer who left a spoor in my path. I was so unbearably sophisticated, convinced I could reconfigure the Tracy/Hepburn magic, so glib and airy-fairy that my shit didn't stink. For a time I even began to question my life with Roger, and Puck as well, as being perhaps too bourgeois for words.

None of the scripts got made, of course. I was tossed on my ass as a loser and a failure, unable to get my calls returned, no matter how desperately I courted the assistants of assistants. I fell into a wrongheaded love affair with a hustler—literally, the fifty-bucks-a-pop variety—which reminds me, I never paid the debt to the starlet for Puck's shots, which would have been a lot better use of the money. Within a few weeks the hustler had sucked all my marrow and moved on. I careened through a year of near-breakdown, writing plays but mostly whining, and nearly driving Roger away in the process.

Yet we never stopped taking that evening walk, along the rim of the hill that led from Kings Canyon to Queens, Puck rooting ahead of us through the chaparral. I'm not quite sure how he managed to serve two masters, but was clearly far too well-bred to choose sides. We simply represented different or-bits, centered of course on him. I was the one who sat at the desk while he slept at my feet all day, and Roger the one who came home at six, sending him into paroxysms of excited barking. The late-night walk was a threesome, no hierarchy of power. I'm not saying it kept Roger and me together, all on its own, but the evening stroll had about it a Zen calm—so many steps to the bower of jacarandas at Queens Road, so many steps home.

I remember the first time the dog howled, when a line of fire trucks shrilled up the canyon to try to cut off a brushfire. Puck threw back his head and gave vent to a call so ancient, so lupine really, that it seemed to have more in common with the ravening of fire and the night stalk of predators than with the drowsy life of a house pet. The howl didn't erupt very often; usually it was kicked off by a siren or a chorus of baying coyotes up-canyon quarreling with the moon. And it was clear Puck didn't like to have us watch him when he did it, especially to laugh or applaud him. He'd been seized by a primal hunger, sacred even, and needed to be alone with it. Usually it lasted no more than a minute, and then he'd be back with us, wagging and begging for biscuits.

We didn't have him fixed, either. More of an oversight than anything else, though I wonder now if it didn't have something to do with the neutering Roger and I had been through during our own years in the closet. It meant of course that Puck could be excruciatingly randy. His favorite sexual activity was to hump our knees as we lay in bed reading at night, barking insistently if we tried to ignore his throbbing need. We more or less took turns, Roger and I, propping our knees beneath the comforter so Puck could have his ride. He never actually came, not a full load, though he dribbled a lot. I can't say if all this made him more of a gay dog or not.

Except for that nightly erotic charge he never actually jumped up on people, though he could be a handful when friends came over, turning himself inside out to greet them. And for some reason—probably having to do with the turkey and ham on the buffet—he loved parties, the bigger the better, wagging about from guest to guest all evening, one eye always on the kitchen and the disposition of scraps.

A dog's life, to be sure, but not really a life destined for heroics—huddling beside a wounded hiker to keep him warm or leading smoke-blinded tenants from a conflagrated house. That was all right: heroics weren't part of the contract. I once read about a woman in England who applied for a seeing-eye dog but specified that she wanted one who'd flunked. She wasn't *very* blind, you see, and besides she wasn't very good at passing tests herself. So she wanted a sort of second-best companion to muck along with her, doing the best they could.

My sentiments exactly. I wasn't planning on any heroics in my life either. Puck didn't have to save me and Roger, and we didn't have to save him.

Except he did, save us in the end. I don't see how he could have known about the insidious onset of AIDS, the dread and the fevers, the letting of blood by the bucketful for tests that told us nothing, and finally Roger's exile to UCLA Medical Center, sentence without parole. I suppose Puck must've picked up on my own panic and grief, suddenly so ignored that he probably counted himself lucky to get his supper. I had no expectations of him except that he stay out of the way. It was then that I began to let him out on his own late at night.

Nobody liked that. Several about-to-be-former friends thought it was terribly irresponsible of me, leaving the dog prey to the coked-up traffic that thundered up the hill when the clubs on the Strip closed. Not to mention those coyotes traveling in packs from trash barrel to trash barrel. They didn't understand how rigorously I'd admonish Puck that he not go far and come back straightaway, any more than they understood that they were just displacing the helplessness they felt over Roger's illness. One time Roger's brother had a near-foaming tantrum about the sofa in the living room, grimy and doubtless flea-infested from years of dog naps. "You can't expect people to visit," Sheldon sputtered. "It smells like a kennel in here."

No, it actually smelled like death, when you came right down to it. The whole house did. And frankly, the only one who could live with the stink, the battlefield stench of shallow unmarked graves, was Puck. Those who proposed re-upholstery as a general solution to keeping death away stopped in less and less, good riddance. The ones who thought we were letting the dog run wild were lucky I didn't sic him on them. Only I really understood, because I saw it happen, how Puck would temper his huge ebullience if Roger was feeling a little fragile. Always there to be petted, sometimes a paw on your knee to nudge you into it.

The world narrowed and narrowed, no end to the tunnel and thus no pin of light in the distance. Not to say there weren't precious months, then weeks, then days, that still had the feel of normalcy. I'd cook up a plate of spaghetti, and we'd sit in the dining room talking of nothing at all, just glad to have a lull in the shelling. And we both looked over one night and saw Puck sitting at attention on his haunches, the sable sheen of his coat set off by the flash of white at his heart, head lifted as if on show, utterly still. In all probability he was just waiting for leftovers. But Roger, bemused and quietly beaming with pride, studied the pose and finally said, "Puck, when did you get to be such a noble beast?"

We both laughed, because we knew we'd had nothing to do with it. But from that point on, Noble Beast became the changeling's nickname. If he took the pose beside you, it meant he wanted his chest scratched. Nothing dramatic, you understand, but somehow Puck came to represent the space left over from AIDS. With no notion of the mortal sting that shaped our human doggedness, he managed to keep the real world ambient, the normal one. Filling it edge to edge with what the thirteenth century divine, Duns Scotus, called "thisness." There gets to be almost nothing more to say about the daily choke of drugs to get down, the nurses streaming in to start the IV drips, the numbing reports to the scatter of family and those few friends who've squeaked through with you. Nothing more to say except what the dog brings in, even if it's mostly fleas.

That last morning, when the home nurse woke me at seven to say it was very bad, Roger virtually comatose, no time to wait for our noon appointment at UCLA, I leapt out of bed and got us out of there in a matter of minutes. I don't remember the dog underfoot. Only holding Roger upright as we staggered down the steps to the car, talking frantically to keep him conscious. Puck would've been perched on the top step watching us go, he'd done that often enough. But I don't really know what he *saw,* any more than I knew what Roger saw—what dim nimbus of light still lingered with one eye gone blind overnight six months before, the other saved by a thrice-daily blast of Acyclovir, but even it milked over with a cataract.

He died that night, and the weeks after are a cataract blur of their own. Somebody must've fed the dog, for I have the impression of him wandering among the houseful of family and friends, trying to find someone who'd lead him to Rog. When we brought home from the hospital the last pitiful overnight bag, the final effects as it were, and Roger's father shook out the maroon coat sweater and put it on for closeness' sake, Puck began to leap up and down, dancing about the old man in a circle, barking deliriously. Because he could still smell life in there.

Have we gotten sentimental yet—gone over the edge? I spent that first annihilating year of grief dragging myself out of bed because somebody had to let the dog out, writing so I wouldn't have to think. I can't count the times when I'd crawl under one of the tables where Puck lay sleeping, to hold him so I could cry. He grumbled at being invaded, but his growl was pretty *pro forma.* And somewhere in there I started to talk to him, asking him if he missed Rog, wondering out loud how we were ever going to get through this—daft as a Booth cartoon. He sat unblinking, the Noble Beast as listener.

I don't know when it started, his peculiar habit of barking whenever visitors would leave. He'd always barked eruptively in greeting, whenever he heard the footfall of a friend coming up the stairs outside. But this new bark was something far more urgent, angry and troubled, a peal of warning, so that I'd have to drag him back by the collar as one bewildered friend or another made his drowned-out goodnights. "He doesn't like people to leave," I'd tell them, but I didn't understand for months what he was warning them of: that if they left they might not come back, might get lost the way Roger did. Don't leave, stay here, I'll keep you safe as I keep this man. Meaning me.

Still, he got over the grief sooner than I, testimony to his blessed unconsciousness of death. He became himself again, inexhaustible, excited anew by the dailiness of life. I'm afraid I'd aged much more than he, maybe twenty years for the twenty months of Roger's illness. Puck was just six, a warrior still in his prime. I had to do a fair bit of traveling there for a while, the self-appointed seropositive poster child. And Puck would lie waiting under my desk, caretaken by Dan the house-sitter, ears perked at every sound outside in case it was me returning from the wars.

Like Argos, Odysseus' dog. Twenty years old and shunted aside because he was too frail to hunt anymore. Waiting ten years for his master's return from Troy, and the only one in the palace to recognize the king beneath the grizzle and the tattered raiment. The earliest wagging tail in literature, I believe. There was no shyness in that time of gods and heroes when it came to the sentiments of reunion, let alone what loyalty meant. So I would come home from ten days' book-touring, from what seemed a mix of overweening flattery and drive-time call-ins from rabid Baptists who painted me as the incarnation of Satan; I would return scarcely able to say who the real Monette was, indeed if there was one anymore—till Puck ran out to welcome me.

Around that time I began to feel ready to risk the heart again, I who hadn't really had a date in fifteen years. I "lingered hopefully" (to quote the advice that Stevie Smith's lion aunt read out to her niece from the lovelorn column); lingered hopefully, I say, at the edges of various parties, in smoke-filled *boîtes,* even at rallies and protests, looking to connect. Held back by my own sero status as much as anything, unsure if I wanted to find only another positive, or whether a lucky negative might rescue my brain from the constant pound of AIDS.

I was on a stationary bike at the gym, pumping hard and going nowhere (too sweaty to be lingering hopefully), when a young man of thirty or so came up and stood before me, catching my eye with a bright expectant nod. "Excuse me," he said, "but aren't you Edmund White?"

"Not exactly," I retorted. Yet it was such an eccentric pickup line that I let him pick me up with it. At least he was literate. I waxed quite eloquent about Ed's work, was quite modest about my own, and gave no further thought to the not-so-subtle omen that the young man might have no interest whatever in Monette, real or otherwise. After all, if you want to read *Moby Dick, Jane Eyre* just won't do.

A few nights later he came over for Chinese takeout. And took an immediate dislike to Puck—nothing personal, he assured me, all dogs really—especially not wanting to sit on the dog-haired sofa in his ice-cream linen trousers. Puck returned the compliment in spades, grumping beneath the coffee table, growling when the young man came too close to me. I apologized for Puck's ragged manners, then deftly turned the subject to AIDS, my own reality check.

His green eyes lit on me. "There's no reason for anyone to die of that," he observed. "All you have to do is take care of yourself. People who die of it, that's just their excuse."

Too stunned or too Episcopalian to savage my first date since puberty, I left the growling to Puck. But I only barely restrained his collar when the young man left, wincing palely at the mastiff shrill of the dog's goodbye.

Stevie had it easier all around. He liked Puck's attitude from the first, recognizing a certain orneriness and perversity that neatly matched his own. If you wanted Puck to come over to you, it did no good to call unless you had a biscuit in hand. In fact I had been bribing him so long—a Meaty Bone to get him outside, another to bring him in—that he acted as if you must be crazy to order him around without reward. It had to be *his* idea to clamber up on the bed or play with a squeak toy. With the latter he wasn't into give-and-take in any case, but snatched it out of your hand and disappeared with it into his lair. Needless to say, "fetch" wasn't in his vocabulary.

I had to learn to back off and feint with Stevie, three months' uncertain courtship. He'd never really made the couple thing work before, and couldn't imagine starting now in the midst of a minefield. It required the barricades for us, going to Washington in October with ACT UP to take over the FDA. A sobbing afternoon spent lurching down the walkways of the quilt, a candle march along the reflecting pool with a hundred thousand others. Then massing at FDA headquarters in Maryland, not even dawn yet (and I don't do mornings), standing groggily with Vito Russo as we briefed the press. A standoff most of the day, squads of cops huddled as if at a doughnut stand, trying not to arrest us.

And then a small gang of six, all from L.A., found a lacuna in the security. Somebody smashed a ground-floor window, and the L.A. guerrillas poured in—Stevie bringing up the rear, impish as Peter Pan himself. When they dragged him out in handcuffs twenty minutes later, the look that passed between us was the purest sign I could've wanted of his being in love with life again. Civil disobedience as aphrodisiac. Within a day we were lovers for real, unarmed and no turning back.

But he wouldn't move in, not to my place. I thought it had to do with the freight of memory, too much Roger wherever you looked. Then I understood how determined he was not to turn the house on Kings Road into a sickroom again—a sickroom that only went one way, to the hospice stage and the last racked weeks. From his own falling numbers, and then the bone-chilling arrival of the first lesion on the roof of his mouth, he knew he'd be out of here sooner than I. (Unless of course I got hit by the bus that seronegatives were forever invoking to prove we were all a hairsbreadth away from the grave—a bus that was always as far behind schedule as we were ahead of it.)

So Stevie began the search for an apartment near me in West Hollywood. Even then we almost broke up a couple of times. He was too far sunk in the quicksand of the endless doctoring, too out of control to be loved. He savaged me one day, calling me blameless even as the arrows found the target of my heart, then fell into a three-day silence. To Victor, who served as go-between in the pained negotiation that followed, he declared: "Why am I breaking up with Paul? I don't know. I like his dog too much."

Oh, that. The fear of getting too attached to the things of life, till you sometimes feel you're better off lying in bed with the shades all down, no visitors welcome. And NO GIFTS, as the invitations all pointedly warn whenever we agree to a final birthday or one more Christmas. No more things to add to the pile that will only have to be dispersed, the yard sale more certain than heaven or hell.

Happily, Puck and I won out. Steve found a place just blocks away, a post-mod apartment behind the Pacific Design Center. And twice a day I'd duck my head under the desk and propose to Puck: "You want to go over to Stevie's?" Then an explosion of barking and dancing, and a long whine of back-seat driving as we headed downhill to Huntley Street. As soon as he saw the house, Puck would leap from the moving car to leave his mark on the bushes, then bark me into the downstairs garage as if I were some recalcitrant sheep.

Stevie was usually in bed, his IVs having doubled, with nothing better to do than flip the remote between one numb banality and the next. Television gave him a place to center his anger, I think, railing at the bad hair and the laugh tracks. A business where he had once commanded so much power— and now his big-screen set practically needed windshield wipers, there was so much spit aimed at it.

But his face would brighten like a kid's when Puck tore in and bounded onto the bed, burrowing in and groaning with pleasure as Stevie gave him a scratch. "Puck, you're better than people," he'd praise the beast—a real irony there, for the beast preferred people to dogs any day.

As for sentiment, Stevie carried that off with the effortless charm he once squandered on agents and actors and network VPs. We'd be driving to one of the neighborhood restaurants, pass a street dog rooting for garbage, and Steve would give an appraising look and wonder aloud: "You think he's a friend of Puck's?" No response required from me, as the answer was quickly forthcoming: "I think he is."

In fact, the question went international quite soon thereafter. With so much medicine required on a daily basis, bags of IV drugs to be kept chilled, the only way we could travel was by ship. So we cruised through the final year—Monte Carlo to Venice, Tahiti to Bora Bora, Greece and Turkey—spending the fat disability checks from Columbia.

One day ashore in the Iles des Saintes, a necklace of pirate lagoons below Guadeloupe, we motorbiked to the highest point, winding through denuded fields, for goats were the main livestock here. We sat on a wall of mortared conchs and looked out to sea. It was one of those moments you want to stop time, knowing what torments lie waiting at journey's end. From a shack behind us emerged a gaggle of children, and behind them a tiny black goat still wobbly on its kid legs. No way could it keep up with the children running downhill to the harbor. So the goat crossed the road to where we were, made for Stevie and butted his knee, so gently it might have been a kiss. Then did it again.

"Friend of Puck's, definitely," Stevie observed with a laugh. A laugh fit for paradise, utterly careless, a holiday from dying.

So what do you carry with you once you have started to leave the world behind? Stevie was right that last Monday in the ICU: he was never going to see Puck again. Didn't even have a chance to say goodbye, except inside. For his part Puck made his own bewildered peace, still tearing into Huntley Street as we packed and gave away one man's universe of things, the beast still hoping against hope that Stevie himself would walk in any minute.

I understand that a housedog is yet another ridiculous privilege of having means in a world gone mad with suffering. I've seen the scrawny dogs that follow refugees around in war after pointless war. The dogs have disappeared from the starvation camps of Somalia, long since eaten in the dogless camps of Laos and Bangladesh. There is nothing to pet in the end. Perhaps it is worse than sentimental, the direst form of denial, to still be weeping at dog stories. But I admit it. Puck has gone gray in the face now, stiff in the legs when he stands, and I am drawn to stories about dogs who visit nursing homes and hospitals, unafraid of frailty and the nearness of death. Dogs, in a word, who don't flunk.

And I weep these incorrigible tears. Two years ago I was in a posh photo gallery in New York with a friend, and we asked to see the Wegmans. I maintained a rigorous connoisseur's posture, keeping it all high-toned, for there were those who were very suspicious of the popularity of Man Ray, the supreme model in Wegman's canine fantasias. There was a general wariness that Wegman's audience might be more interested in dogs than art. In my case doubly so, since to me at least Puck could have been Man Ray's twin. Same color, same shape, same humanness.

Now of course Man Ray was gone, and though he'd been replaced in the studio by the sleek and estimable Fay—no mean model herself—prices for a vintage Man had gone through the roof. Anyway, this curatorial assistant, very 57th Street, brought out of a drawer with white gloves three big Polaroids of Man. In one the dog was stretched on his back with his paws up; no gimmicks or costume accessories here, just a dog at rest. You could tell he was old from the shiver of gray on his snout. I found it so unbearably moving that I choked on tears and could not look at another.

After Stevie was buried, I figured Puck and I were set for twilight, seven years for every twelvemonth, a toss-up still as to who'd go first. We didn't plan on letting anyone else in. Not depressed or even defeated yet—just exhausted, hearts brimful already with seized days and a sort of Homeric loyalty, we shared a wordless language and had no expectations. Like the old man and his dog in DeSica's masterpiece *Umberto D,* who cannot save each other but can't leave either. They'd rather starve together.

Then I met Winston. It was a bare two months since Steve had died, and Victor and I had just returned from three weeks' melancholy touring in Europe, weeping in cathedrals so to speak. I recall telling Victor on the flight home that I could probably still connect with someone, but only if that someone could handle the steamship-load of AIDS baggage I carried with me. Somehow Winston could juggle it with his own, or perhaps the risk and intoxication of love made even the dead in our arms lighter. By Christmas we were lovers, and Puck couldn't help but give us his blessing, so showered was he by Winston with rubber bones and pull toys: "This dog has got nothing to play with!"

The dog was not the only one. And because there is never enough time anymore, by mid-January we were deep into the chess match of Winston's move into Kings Road. Just one small problem, really—a four-year-old boxer called Buddy. He'd grown up on a ranch, free to run and in titular charge of a barnful of horses and a tribe of cats. The first meeting of our two unfixed males wasn't promising. Buddy jumped on Puck right off, sending the two of them into a whirlwind ball of snarling and gnashing, leaving Winston and me no choice but to wade in and pull them apart. Buddy was clearly the aggressor here, but then we were on his territory.

The situation didn't improve when Buddy came to stay at
Kings Road. Puck was outraged that his slumbering twilight
had been invaded. He stuck to his lairs and growled with ferocious menace if Buddy came anywhere near. In fact, if we
weren't absolutely vigilant we had a sudden dogfight on our
hands. There was nothing for it but to separate them at opposite ends of the house, the doors all closed. It was like a French
farce, with the constant flinging and slamming of doors, and
enough entrances and exits to rival the court of the Louis.

You get used to compromises when everyone you know
is dying. It was clear that Buddy was a pussycat at heart, his
gentle spirit every bit as benign as Puck's lab side, except when
they were together. And Buddy was meticulously trained as
well, as rigorous as a Ballanchine dancer, responding with in-
finite grace to all of his master's commands. Responding to
food alone, Puck didn't know quite what to make of the military precision of his housemate.

Puck was fed on the front porch, Buddy in the back yard.
It was no more peculiar in its way than families who can't
stand one another, sitting silent at the dinner table, invisible
lines drawn. If Winston and I hadn't been able to laugh about
it, I'm not sure it could have gone on so long. But by April
he had bitten the bullet and had Buddy fixed, though we were
warned it could take six months for the pugnacity around Puck
to abate. Puck's balls followed on the chopping block in June,
since the vet assured me Puck would have fewer problems
aging, less chance of tumors if he were fixed.

They didn't really seem any different that summer, except
that Puck wouldn't hump our knees with the same rollicking
passion. He humped all right, but it seemed more of an after-
thought, a memory trace, over in a matter of seconds. I didn't
have much leisure to notice, frankly, with my own numbers
falling precipitously and three ribs broken from taking a dive
off a trotting horse. The walls of AIDS were closing in, no

matter how tortuous my progress through the drug underground, scoring the latest miracle. It was all I could do not to drown in my own panic, or take it out on Winston. My attitude toward the dogs was more impatient than ever, but Puck had been there before. There were times when dogs just had to be dogs—no neediness, please, and no misbehaving. The merest tick became a problem I couldn't handle.

By the end of summer I'd started to run daily fevers— 99.5 at five P.M., like clockwork. My T-cells continued to tumble, under a hundred now. Winston had to fly up to Seattle over Labor Day weekend to visit his former lover, John, who'd taken a very bad turn. It was the first time I'd had the two dogs by myself. All I really wanted to do was sit at the word processor, only three or four pages to go in *Becoming a Man*. And it seemed I spent all day opening and closing doors, a solo performer in a farce.

Finally I'd had it. I called Buddy in from the bedroom, Puck from the fleabag sofa. I sat them down at opposite ends of the study, threatening them direly if they dared make a move toward each other. They both blinked at me as I lectured them: this separate-but-equal shit had got to stop. "Now lie down and be good boys," I commanded with a final flourish.

And they did. Puzzled, I am sure, by the heat of my remark.

There were still rough edges, of course. Now that they managed to be together without attacking, they began to steal toys from each other, swooping in and snatching, the growls just short of a major explosion. The problem was, Puck didn't know how to play—he was as loath to share as a bully in kindergarten or the spoiled brat who takes his baseball home so nobody else can enjoy it. The toys would pile up in his lair, guarded like meat. Buddy—such a prince—was the one who was eager to play in earnest, and yet he'd yield to Puck and forgo the tearing around the house he loved—turning the other cheek, so to speak, rather than bristling. It may have been the loss of balls that let it happen, but clearly Buddy preferred to have a friend than to be on top.

Gradually Puck learned to give a little back, permitting Buddy to do his racing about with a mauled stuffed Dumbo in his mouth, while Puck stood ground and barked. But if Buddy gets credit for teaching Puck the rudiments of play, the pedagogy went the other way when it came to making noise. When Buddy first arrived he didn't make a peep, never having been needed as a watchdog at the ranch. Thus he'd watch with a certain fascination as Puck, alert to every sound outside, especially the arrival of delivery men, ran to the front door bellowing doom. It took a fair amount of time for Buddy to get the hang of it—a softer bark in any case, here too letting Puck be the lead singer—but now they both leap up clamoring, barreling by one another as they scramble to investigate.

In fact it's Puck who's had to yield in the watchdog department. After all, Buddy's hearing is finer, his high-pointed ears like radar. Puck's has dimmed in his twelfth year, so he doesn't quite catch the slam of every car door. More often now Buddy's the one who pricks to the sound of something out there, the first to woof, so that Puck's scramble to join the fray is an act of following.

And Puck has been more than a little grateful to turn the rat chores over to Buddy. We have brown field rats, not so horrible as the gray vermin that haunt the docks and garbage dumps of the world. Sometimes one gets in because the kitchen door is open to the back yard, to give the dogs access. A couple of times Puck and I have surprised a rodent in the kitchen, and I shriek and Puck barks, and somehow the freaked-out rat scoots away.

But Buddy's a ratter. He sniffs them out and waits for them to make their move from under the stove or the washing machine. He'll wait for hours if necessary. And when the rodent makes a dash for the kitchen door, Buddy's on him—unafraid to clamp his jaws around the squirming intruder and give him a bad shake. He doesn't kill them, just scares the bejesus out of them. If I were a rat I would not be coming back soon. And since I can't stand to trap them anymore—that awful springing snap as the trip-arm breaks a leg or neck—I much prefer the Buddy method of pest control.

It would be too simple to call them brothers now, these two dogs, too anthropomorphic by half. Each has retained the marks and idiosyncracies of his breed quite distinctly. Buddy is what is called a "flashy fawn," because all four paws are white as well as his breastplate and a marvelous zigzag just behind his ears. He can't stand getting wet, doesn't even like to be in the garden after it's been watered, practically walking on tiptoe. While Puck no longer dives into the pool as he used to, swimming laps with Roger, water is still his element. On a very hot day he'll still step down in and dog-paddle in a tight circle to cool off.

Not brothers then, but comrades. Like any other dogs they sleep more than anything else, but sometimes now they do it flank to flank, almost curled about each other. When they sit on their haunches side by side in the kitchen doorway, lingering hopefully for biscuits, they are most definitely a pair. (Puck taught Buddy to beg, by the way, a serious breach in his training.) When they go outside together, Buddy knows he can go no further than the edge of the terrace, not down the steps. Puck on the other hand sprawls himself on the landing at the top of the stairs, one step down from the terrace, his lifelong perch for overseeing the neighborhood. Thus Buddy stands above Puck, though one would be hard put to say who's taking care of whom.

That they look after each other is clear. It's an act of faith among conservative zoologists that there's no homosex in the

animal world. Gay is a human orientation, period. But just as
I've come to understand, late in my own dog years, that being
gay is a matter of identity much larger than carnality, I don't
think the mating instinct is all the story. What the two dogs
have is an easy sort of intimacy, the opposite of straight men.
Thus they sniff each other's buttholes as casually as men shake
hands. Not gay then, exactly, even though both have grown
up surrounded by a tribe of us: call them different, that comes
closest. As if being together has changed them so that they've
become more than themselves—a continuum of eccentricities
traded off and mimicked, grounded by their willingness to be
tamed, loyal before all else. Not unlike Winston and me, and
we're as gay as they come.

Meanwhile, twilight deepens. The dogs whoop with delight when Ande the nurse comes to call, once a week these
days so I can get my IV dose of Amphotericin. They do not
see her as a chill reminder of my sickness, any more than I do.
We humans sustain this life as best we can, propelled by the
positive brand of denial, the nearest approximation we can
make to the bliss of dogs and their mortal ignorance. Thus I
can watch Puck age and feel it tear at me, while he can't watch
me dwindle or even see the lesions. Somehow it makes him
wiser than I am, for all my overstuffed brains, book-riddled
and smart to a fault.

We go along as we always have, a household of four instead of two. Every few weeks Puck and I cross Kings Road
to visit Mrs. Knecht, our neighbor who lost her husband in
'85 to a sudden heart attack. She endures in her eighties, a
tribute to her Austrian stalwartness, her family wiped out in
the camps. Assaulted by the indignities of age, Mrs. Knecht
doesn't have a lot of pleasures anymore, but Puck is one. I'm
terrified that he'll knock her down when he barrels into her
house, that he'll take her hand off when she feeds him biscuits.
But that is what she likes best about him, I think, his indomita-

ble eagerness, his stallion force. Mrs. Knecht is our good deed, Puck's and mine, but also serving to remind all three of us that life goes on among the loyal.

Nights we stay up later than Buddy and Winston, a couple of hours at least. Buddy curls in his basket under the bedroom window, and Winston like Roger sleeps without pills, deeper than I ever get. I can't really say that Puck stays up with me as I potter around in the still of the night. He sleeps too, though always near me, and he would call it keeping me company if he had words. All he knows is, nothing is likely at this hour to bother us or require his vigilance. It will go on like this forever, as far as Puck can see. For his sake I try to see no further, relishing these hours out of time.

It has already been decided: if I go first Winston has promised to care for him, to keep what's left of the family together. If Puck goes first, perhaps a painless shot to end some arthritic misery, I promise nothing. The vets will tell you, there are suicides in the parking lot after the putting down of pets. For some it's the last last straw.

But for tonight I'm glad we have endured together and, as they say in the romance genre, lived to love again. We will not be returning from Troy, either of us, but meanwhile we are one another's link to the best of the past, a matter of trust and bondedness that goes all the way back to prehistory. One of us is descended from wolves; one of us knows he's dying. Together we somehow have the strength to bear it, tonight at least, when the moon is down and no creature howls. What we dream is exactly the same, of course, that nothing will change.

At two A.M. he whimpers at the door to go out, and I let him go. Usually he's back in half an hour, but you never know what will take him further, what trail will beckon him up through the chaparral. He knows me too well. That I'll wait up all night if necessary till he comes panting home. That even if I rail at him like a crabby parent, he'll still get a biscuit before the lights go out. Because all that matters to either of us is that the other one's still here—fellow survivors of so much breakage to the heart, not a clue when the final siren will sound. But guarding the world for dear life anyway, even as it goes. Noble beast.

GERT

"DOES IT GO TOO FAST?" I asked her.

The three of us were sitting in a booth at '21,' Gert and Roger and I, having supper after the theater. Robert Benchley's booth, as a matter of fact, a spitball's throw from the downstairs bar. Gert had such a vivid memory of the bar's heyday that she could people the room with the regulars, Moss Hart to Cole Porter, transporting us back to a time of effortless glamour. No matter that Roger or even I didn't recognize half the names. I at least could keep up with her — *Wasn't he a set designer? Didn't she used to sing in musicals?* — enough to get her going and fill us in with stories fit for Damon Runyon. It astonished her how little the young remembered about the glory days of Broadway. How could it be — these giants who bestrode the glittering streets outside, the toasts of the town — how could they have vanished so?

At first she didn't appear to understand my question. "Does what go too fast?" She took a last delirious puff from an unfiltered Camel — oh, how she could smoke — and I backed off a little, thinking perhaps the question had been too forward. "Oh, you mean *life*," she replied with a dawning smile, stubbing out the cigarette. "Not at all. It seems just as long as it ought to be. Well, the anniversaries maybe—they come round faster and faster every year. But don't worry, you're not going to feel you haven't had enough. Why are you thinking about *that?*"

Genuinely puzzled, a frown creasing the great wrinkled terrain of her face. A cross between Lillian Hellman and W. H. Auden, with the same fissured map that hid nothing of the cram of experience, though more lovely than either. Life drunk to the lees, plus five thousand cartons of Camels.

She would have been seventy-five then, because there were about forty years between us, and I retorted haltingly, "But I'm thirty-four already, and I've . . . I don't know, gotten such a late start." I meant in the theater, though the subtext was still all those wasted years in the closet.

Gert guffawed delightedly, sharing the laugh with Roger. "But you're still a baby," she chided me, yet somehow without a shred of contempt. "You've got all the time in the world. I didn't even hit my stride till I was fifty-five."

I remember feeling comforted by that—an antidote to the relentlessness of the California youth-cult, the unwritten rule that put a writer out to pasture at forty, no longer hip. Or the equally sinister look that went right through you on Santa Monica Boulevard from the buffed pups of West Hollywood who never seemed to age at all. Their arms got bigger, their shoulders and chests bulging with good health, but they never crossed the border into a full-grown man's experience. There were no models for getting old anyway, not there among the clattering palms and the hydrocarbon smut of perfect weather. Old meant Palm Springs, tired old queens and their daiquiris, and the young avoided them assiduously, as if age itself were catching.

Thus did Gert become my role model for growing old alive. She was also my first lesbian, the first I really knew—

though she kept to a rigorous code of silence when it came to the proclivities of the theater girls of her generation. I don't suppose she ever said the word directly, certainly not by way of self-identification, but that was all right with me. I wouldn't make her say it out loud, as long as she taught me the code. Besides, I was out enough for both of us. Of course I knew lesbians in Boston, writers and community activists, but these were still the years of separatist growing pains, a gulf of apprehension and mistrust between the men and women of the tribe. Still trapped by one another's stereotypes, and the past a matter of mostly shadows. Not enough sages and grandparents.

I met her in the most improbable place, at a Canton graduation. This was a *girls'* school graduation, virginal to a fault, austere as a Shaker hymn. Afterward on the lawn, the faculty mingled with the girls' families, picking at the lobster buns and petit fours that seemed to grow staler and more rancid by the year, an afternoon tea out of a cryogenics vault. Gert—Miss Gertrude Macy—the maiden great-aunt of one of my students, was sitting knock-kneed on one of the grisly folding chairs, still cobwebbed from storage, that cluttered the lawn behind the library.

I was graciously introduced as the school poet. "I had no idea there were still poets around," remarked Miss Macy in her gravelly voice. "How encouraging."

It was only a moment before I was sitting cross-legged beside her chair, trying to hide from my dreary graduation duties in the shade of Miss Macy's presence. It turned out she had worked in the theater all her life, serving as stage manager and general factotum for Miss Katharine Cornell's company. Unarguably, Cornell was the leading lady of American theater in the time between the wars. Gert started with her in 1928, through the yearly triumphs in New York—*Candida, The Barretts of Wimpole Street, Saint Joan, Romeo and Juliet, Antigone*—and then when the season was over, going on the road with the touring company.

I was the perfect audience for the backstage version of all
of this. I'd grown up bitten by the theater, done my share of
teeth-jarring overacting while in college, and still went faith-
fully to the Boston tryouts of everything. I had even seen Miss
Cornell on stage in her last tour, a two-character performance
with Brian Aherne called *Dear Liar,* being the letters of Shaw
and Mrs. Patrick Campbell. Not much of a play at all, really,
with just the two of them standing at lecterns. And Gert would
tell me later how grueling that tour was, Cornell but a ghost
of the diva she had been. But at least I'd been in the presence,
and so could imagine the Kit Cornell who swept through
Gert's marvelous stories.

One year they were on their way to Seattle, the whole
company on a train, *The Barretts* I think. It's difficult to imagine today how profound the excitement was, when a star of
Cornell's magnitude came to the provinces, bag and baggage,
a genuine New York production in tow. Alas, there was late
spring snow in the mountains, and the train got mired. No
way were they going to make Seattle for opening night, that
very evening. Gert telegraphed ahead to cancel the first performance.

They pulled into Seattle about ten hours late, exhausted
and chilled. The theater owner met them coming off the train,
as the sets and costumes were being unloaded from boxcars.
He announced to Gert that the audience was waiting at the
theater in their seats. By now it was ten or eleven P.M., and it
would take hours to put up the set and light it. They simply
couldn't perform tonight.

But the audience wouldn't leave, no matter how many
announcements were made, even the offer of a special performance at the end of the run. They just sat there politely in
their evening clothes. And because Kit and the others grew up
in a time when the show just *had* to go on, the curtain went
up a little before dawn, transporting them all back to Wimpole
Street in the 1830s. A thrilling performance, according to Gert,

though it could hardly have been a bust with such an amazing prelude. The burghers of Seattle clapped their gloves off.

Gert had known everyone, from Olivier to Brando, the latter playing Marchbanks to Kit's umpteenth revival of *Candida*. They didn't really know any *movie* stars to speak of, unless they had acted first on the stage. Hollywood was so far beneath the notice of Miss Cornell and her fellow stage immortals. All her life she turned down script after script, chance after chance to preserve herself on celluloid. But to her generation Hollywood was the opposite of "legitimate," not even close to what they in the theater called acting. Thus there is scarcely any record at all of the great lady's work, except for a moment's cameo in *Stage Door Canteen*, undertaken for patriotic reasons.

Gert wasn't so much of a snob herself, and admitted to an unapologetic fanship. She was breathless the day Olivier brought his new wife, Vivien Leigh, backstage to meet Cornell. But most overwhelming of all was the unannounced appearance of Garbo in the aisle seat in Row H, the seat beside her reserved for her fur coat. Remember, Gert reminded me, warming to her favorite anecdote, this was at a time when Garbo was mythic, thousands of women in New York affecting the slouch hat and the hooded look of the otherworldly star. Alerted to her presence, Gert and the rest of the company peeked through the crack in the curtains, gasping.

Then Miss Cornell herself appeared and demanded to know what the ruckus was. She took a quick peek and declared the woman in Row H nothing but a wannabe (or whatever they called them then). And besides, she declared imperiously, who *cared* about Garbo and all that nonsense. Places please, we have a show to put on!

As *The Barretts* reached its climax, Gert put in a fast call to L.A., to a publicist she knew who'd worked with Garbo. "Do you know where she is right this minute?" asked Gert when he took the call. As a matter of fact, he said, he had no idea at all, for Garbo had disappeared from a movie set about three days before, leaving the whole of the glitter kingdom in the lurch. Accustomed to such behavior by now, the studio bit its nails and waited.

When Kit came offstage at last, with a dozen curtain calls and an armload of roses, Gert confronted her triumphantly: it *was* the real thing out there. Airily Kit dismissed the news and made for her dressing room. Gert fumed. Then five minutes later the Swedish diva herself appeared at the stage door, shy and practically muffled in her fox collar, pulled in like a turtle. "Miss Garbo to see Miss Cornell," mumbled that unmistakable voice. A stunned Gert stepped forward and led legend to meet legend.

Kit wouldn't let Gert come in with Garbo. Gert paced impatiently, and about ten minutes later Kit stuck her head out of the dressing room, sweetly ordering her to take Guthrie over to '21' for supper. Guthrie McClintic was Kit's husband and director for forty years, a gay man, as I later found out. Sent off like children, Gert and Guthrie ordered stiff martinis and caviar at the restaurant, defying Kit's rule that her guests could order anything on the menu *except* caviar, which even she with all her extravagance thought too dearly priced.

When Gert and Guthrie came lurching home to Beekman Place, they found that Kit had brought Garbo to the house. The two actresses sat in the parlor before the fire, eating soup and sharing a torn baguette. As Gert came in, Garbo was laughing (Garbo laughs!) and waving her bare feet in the air. "See how big they are!" she announced with glee. "Like a fishwife's!"

This was definitely a story of the Homeric Age, when stars were gods and goddesses. I didn't really think so much at the time about the gay subtext. But for months afterward, whenever I told the story to friends old enough to know the cast of characters, they always interrupted me to say: "Oh yes, Miss Macy—she was Cornell's lover for years. And Guthrie had all the boys." It seemed like a secret that nobody kept. Except it somehow remained unspoken, protected by a wall of glamour that the press wouldn't have dreamed of trying to vault. It was, as I say, a certain understanding—a separate life conducted on the higher slopes of Olympus, underscored by a reflex of discretion. A bohemian aristocracy, if that's not too much of a contradiction in terms.

Gert and I parted fast friends, swearing we'd meet again before the summer waned, but who ever keeps such promises? As it happened, the '76 graduation was my last at Canton Academy. I'd decided I would never be the writer I wanted to be if I stayed in school. I would therefore take a year off and try to write a novel. I'd applied for a grant to see me through, but still hadn't heard about that. Roger said he'd support me, while I swore I'd wait tables if necessary.

I don't recall if Craig and I decided to go to the Vineyard before or after Gert's call. Craig was my closest pal in Boston—met the same night I met Roger two years before, and fascinated like me by the glow of stars and all the attendant tinsel. Of everyone I told, Craig was the one who ate up the story of Garbo in Row H like popcorn.

Anyway, Craig invited me down to Martha's Vineyard for an overnight, to stay with a friend of his youth from Williamstown. I knew Gert had a summer place at the Vineyard, but didn't have the number. Then, just days before we were ready to depart for the Woods Hole ferry to the island, Gert phoned out of the blue. She had a story to tell me, she said, about an extraordinary visitor she'd had at her house on the bluffs of the Hudson, which she'd been in the process of shutting up for the summer before making the trek north to the island. *Garbo,* I blurted in quick reply, and she laughed at my perspicacity. Delighted to hear I was coming over to the Vineyard, she said she'd save the details till then.

Thus Craig and I made our excited way to Gert's place on a drowsy morning in early July. It was hardly bigger than a fisherman's shack—a house for one, make no mistake—and perched on what amounted to a sand bar between the lambent surf of the bay and a reed-rimmed salt pond. So nicely isolated that you could just see the roofpeaks of Gert's near neighbors. Yet we had scarcely entered the little house—shipshape as a captain's quarters, an island all its own—and were still saying hello to Gert when the phone rang.

It was Nancy Hamilton, yet another of the charmed inner circle of Miss Cornell, and like Gert an aging survivor of the golden years. Playwright and lyricist, famous wit, she had given the very best parties in the old days. Kit had left her The Barn on the Vineyard, her last home there, across the pond from Gert's. And now Nancy was calling to inquire suspiciously: Who were those two young men she'd seen driving up the ribbon of beach road to Gert's? She must've been spying with binoculars from the widow's walk to catch a glimpse of us. With a certain malicious glee Gert told Nancy she'd been expecting us, but not a word as to who we were.

We swam in the bay and lay in the sun, while Gert brought us our first bullshot of the day (oh, how she could put away vodka). Then, sitting grandly on her deck in her trademark cobalt-blue-lensed sunglasses, in khaki shorts and an old army shirt, she regaled us with the tale of Garbo's visit. The legendary recluse had been longing to get out of Manhattan, where the weather that June had been unbearably sultry. A mutual friend suggested they spend an afternoon at Gert's place in Sneden's Landing, about fifteen minutes north of the George Washington Bridge. It took a week to coax her, but Garbo finally said yes, adding wearily, "Does she have to know who I am?"

Now don't say anything about her career in pictures, the friend warned Gert. Just a little lunch in the garden, and keep the conversation bland. Gert made sure her collection of little dogs—a veritable pack of Shih-tzus and Pekingese, along with a dimwit Irish setter she'd adopted after a Sneden's neighbor died—stayed inside with the housekeeper. Garbo was offered a sunny spot, a shady spot, the view through the trees to the lordly river below. Nothing was quite right, because she'd left her sweater in the taxi on the way. She fretted about that sweater all afternoon.

I think she affected not to remember the evening she spent with Miss Cornell showing off her big feet—it must have been thirty or forty years ago by then. The more Gert filled in the details, the more did Garbo seem to stiffen and grow aloof. "Not very bright, I'm afraid," Gert told us with keen disappointment. Garbo was wearing a blouse with a hundred buttons all the way up to her chin, and she kept patting at her neck to make sure it didn't show. "Miss Garbo," Gert asked her gently, "why don't you just unbutton your collar and feel the breeze?" After all, they were just three old ladies out on the terrace, no paparazzi for miles around. But no, she stayed buttoned up.

The only other thing I remember from Gert's account of the day Garbo came to lunch happened over the stuffed avocados. Gert was chatting amiably with the mutual friend, and Garbo was staring moodily at the river below, when suddenly she announced, *a propos* of nothing, "I hate it when somebody calls me Gigi." No one had done so. But Gert smiled gamely and observed, "Well, you don't have to worry about that, because everyone in the *world* calls you Garbo." The look on the legend's face just then was a queer mix of offended dignity, as if someone had come too close, and a half-smile of satisfaction, basking in the world's notice.

That was all—no real bullseye anecdotes, no reverberating Garbo lines of the caliber of *I want to be alone* or the first words she ever spoke in pictures, asking for a whiskey in *Anna Christie*. But Craig and I pealed with laughter at every morsel, giddy as a pair of opera queens, as if we were privy to the high jinks of a rare inner circle of our kind. For it didn't need stating aloud here either, that the oh-so-subtle friction between Gert and Garbo was a confrontation of lesbians, a duel over the shadows of the past. Perhaps Craig and I were so ga-ga about the smallest details because these closeted stars were the only kind of role models we had from the past. The work to reclaim our history was only just beginning among the tribe's scholars and chroniclers. In our youth we had to make do with high gossip, and Gert was there for the footnotes.

Craig was more brazen than I that day, oiled by bullshots and bluntly asking, "What was Tallulah like?" Or Julie Harris, whom Gert had produced in *I Am a Camera*. But the story that struck the deepest chord in me was the one about Marlene Dietrich. In '44, Kit and her troupe had volunteered to perform for the Allied troops, a six-month tour of *The Barretts* that took them through Italy and France, sometimes a bare few miles from the fighting. When they finally got to Paris they were wilted and beat, not having had a proper bath in weeks, much less a hot one.

Dietrich, who had never met Cornell, was being put up in the Imperial Suite at the Ritz, vacated by U.S. Navy brass in deference to the supreme entertainer of the Allied forces. Dietrich put in a call to Kit's coldwater hotel and invited her up for a nice, hot bath. Gert went along as an aide-de-camp— damned if she'd be shut out again the way she'd been with Garbo. Dietrich couldn't have been more gracious, leaving the two women alone in a rose marble bath fitted out for a pasha. Kit and Gert luxuriated in the steam and the cloud-like towels. After an hour they dressed and made ready to leave, not wishing to inconvenience the Kraut any further.

But as they were saying goodbye, Dietrich cast a disapproving look at the olive-drab uniforms sported by Kit and Gert. Then she flung open the imperial closet, revealing a whole Savile Row tailor's line of officers' uniforms, one for every branch of the Allied powers, and each one fitted to Dietrich's svelte form. These were the clothes she wore to the front, a sort of reverse mufti, saving the beaded gowns and swan's down coat for performances.

For the next couple of hours the women played dress-up with the military gear—Gert a general, Kit an admiral, Dietrich a Marine commandant, all of them merrily prancing and strutting. I can almost hear their laughter spilling out through the French doors to Place Vendome, the bronze column in the center commemorating a victory over Germans of another era. The Joint Chiefs in drag, as it were.

This was lesbian history of a very high order indeed. The image of the cross-dressed women wouldn't leave me, and was more erotic the more I thought of it. Three weeks later, when I started to work in earnest on my novel, the scene at the Ritz went into the story as part of the legend of my heroine—an aging chanteuse who was clearly based on Dietrich. Yet all my baroque imaginings were pretty weak tea compared to the reality—Dietrich the famous bisexual, notorious by then for the parade of lovers both men and women, the generals and the duchesses. She was more out than almost anyone in Hollywood, so confident was she of her vast unshakable womanhood. The opposite of Kit, with her backstage marriage to Guthrie and her offstage lesbian friends.

Indeed, I could hardly keep them all straight. Once I met an old actor who'd been in several Cornell productions, whose jowls quivered with passion as he waxed about Kit's genius. When the tone had finally lowered to dish, he talked of Gert and Kit as inseparable, then laughed about poor Guthrie, who was ever losing his heart to men who wouldn't love him back—ambitious young actors and hustler types who hung around for a while for the sake of the caviar, leaving Guthrie desolate in the end. Since he knew so much, I asked him offhandedly about this Nancy Hamilton woman, the one with the binoculars.

Ah, but Nancy Hamilton was the second great love of Kit's life—the one who came after Gert. Hearing it, I felt a peculiar defensive pain on Gert's behalf, and couldn't figure out how Gert could stay so close after being supplanted. Her small pavilion among the trees at the edge of the bluff at Sneden's—another house pointedly built for one—was not far from the "big house" where Kit and Guthrie had lived. On Martha's Vineyard Gert had bought the tiny fisherman's shack, after which Kit and Guthrie had grandly acquired the whole nearby point. Perhaps they were all just very grown up, willing to let their relationships elide and change, a loyal troupe no matter who was sleeping with whom. In any case Kit was the queen, the others her ladies-in-waiting. Or maybe *courtiers* is the better word.

I couldn't ever ask Gert to clarify, it would have been overstepping my bounds. She appeared to harbor not the slightest shred of regret or bitterness when it came to Kit's memory. She was keeper of the flame, after all; ever the more so, the more the world forgot. She didn't seem lonely in the least, anymore than she ever seemed regretful. The past had done the best it could with the compromises required to live in it, and there was no purpose in changing the rules now. Let the dead rest, for the theaters they had lit up with their names were all dark anyway.

And yet, if the lavender truth of the past was off-bounds, Gert was no less thrilled to see how the Stonewall generation changed the rules forever. She adored hearing stories of my gay and lesbian friends, for whom being out of the closet was a necessary passage to living life for real. Gert worried about the backlash, having an instinct for the savageries of which religion was capable. Did I really think the Catholics and the Baptists were going to sit back and let our pride go unchallenged? Didn't matter, I said, because we would win. But she wasn't so sure, was still uncomfortable when I spoke of Roger as my lover.

"Can't you just call him your friend?" she wondered aloud on more than one occasion. "Lover sounds so . . ." She paused, at a rare loss for words. "Don't you think friend is more intimate?" As a matter of fact, I do, today. But at the time I liked the shock value of "lover," my whole life having been recast since my long-belated exit from the closet. For a while there, shock was my favorite value. What we did agree about, Gert and I, was the thrill that came with a growing sense of community in the tribe. Indeed, our kind were every-where now, and if Gert was more voyeur than participant in our new-found ubiquity, nevertheless she partook of the pride with a secret satisfaction.

After that midsummer visit with Craig, I only saw her two or three times a year, especially after Roger and I moved to California. Because of her wizened countenance and her bad habits, I never knew if I'd see her again. There was always something poignant about that last wave farewell, as we left each other outside Sardi's and got into separate taxis; an inar-ticulate worry that maybe I hadn't said enough, hadn't probed deep enough. I don't think Gert shared my young man's anxi-ety of incompletion. She was very unsentimental about death, and fierce in her commitment to the right of self-deliverance. You did what you could with the present, just as you did with the past: no regrets. And the last thing anyone needed to stand on was ceremony.

Is that why I gave her so much leeway to counsel me? I remember I sent her my first book of poems, plus a manuscript of my second, a group of dramatic monologues. When I came to see her at Sneden's Landing, she said she had read them all straight through, and managed not to make it sound like going to the dentist. On the contrary, she found them brilliant. Just one thing troubled her: "Exactly who reads them?"

I hastened to reassure her that they were doing quite well among the little magazines (which suddenly sounded positively Lilliputian). And then of course there were my fellow poets, following one another's work—or was it just one another's careers they followed, bristling at the fellowships and sinecures that should have gone to them?

"You should be writing for more than that," she observed.

By which she meant not more rewards, or even the chance of a wider audience, which she knew as well as anyone was mostly a matter of luck. Rather, she sensed a kind of constrictedness and self-absorption in the work, an overdetermined reach—strain, to put it bluntly—for the perfect image. All of which struck fertile ground, for I was beginning to question my own place in the ranks of the silver-tongued poets. The voice wasn't mine anymore.

"You should write a play," said Gert.

But I was writing a novel instead, which I assured her would have the same effect, unfettering my song. She gave me her most enthusiastic encouragement, all too aware that theater was an uphill climb, a world that had undergone sea-changes since the halcyon days of Miss Cornell. I think she was also flattered to hear what an influence she'd had on the *femme d'un certain age* who stood at the center of my story. Gert was certainly first in line to read the galleys when the book reached print at last.

To celebrate, she had me to lunch at the Cosmopolitan Club, a ladies' club straight out of Ruth Draper. A palm-court dining room chockablock with women of a certain age, all of whom wore ice-cream-sundae hats as if in tribute to the Queen Mother. These were the selfsame ladies, Gert confided drolly, who would fill up the matinee performances in the old days; so genteel. Turned out today in a vintage black suit of her own—"my funeral duds," she called them—Gert was distinguishable from the flock only by her blue glasses and bare head. Yet she clearly thought of herself as a kind of renegade among the ladies who lunched: with them but not of them. This was just one of the curious paradoxes of her tightrope walk between bohemia and a minimal gentility.

"And they'd all faint with shock if they read this book of yours," declared Gert. "I was a little shocked myself," she admitted with a deep-throated laugh. "So many sweating bodies!" I think she had rather relished the shock, unaccustomed as she was to sex that was rated X. And then she asked, seeming more fascinated than disapproving: "Does it have to be quite so gay?"

Oh, indeed it did. The gayer the better. I launched into my half-baked credo, invoking the name of Forster, the writer to whom I was most in thrall, and the one who had failed me the most as well. When Forster decided he dare not publish *Maurice*, for fear of the scandal and what his mother would think; when he locked that manuscript in a drawer for fifty years until he died, he silenced much more than himself. He put up a wall that prevented us, his gay and lesbian heirs, from having a place to begin. He had written an unheard-of thing: a queer love story that ended in love fulfilled. But we would have to make do instead with the obsessive torments of *Giovanni's Room* and the broken flowers of Tennessee Williams. It wasn't just my book, but a whole new generation's worth— *Dancer from the Dance, Rubyfruit Jungle, Nocturnes for the King of Naples*—that would speak our passion without any compromise. No matter what our mothers thought.

Gert was unaccustomed to hearing me on a soapbox. She nodded gravely, ceding me the argument, then permitted herself a quick half-smile: "Sometimes you remind me of Shaw, do you know that?" Shaw the haranguer, not Shaw the playwright. And I remember wondering even at the time, between the fingerbowls and the pink parfaits, if I'd gone too far. Did she take it as veiled criticism of her own generation, with its locked drawers and sealed steamer trunks; the truth about whom they really loved held hostage to their need to be discreet before all else? But if it struck her as any sort of accusation, she never let on. She always spurred me forward.

And in return, have I done the wrong thing here, spilling the secret that was second nature to them all, for the sake of a politics of openness of which they could scarcely conceive? I'm pretty sure Gert could have handled any revelation about herself, but she also would have drawn the line at Kit. After all, what do I have for proof but gossip, however high-toned? Hardly the stuff to withstand the scrutiny of history. Instinctively, I feel that the veils shrouding our collective past should be rent, that we must claim as our own the Melvilles and Willa Cathers and Cary Grants. For God's sake, I managed to study Whitman for two years at Yale without it ever being pointed out that he was queer. *Whitman!* (Begging the question of what a dunce I was for not figuring it out myself; but that, as they say, is another story.)

During the next few years I was madly busy, churning out screenplays for Universal with one hand, up half the night writing fiction with the other. It's a wonder I didn't collapse, I was so driven. I certainly wasn't thinking much about what I was writing anymore. It didn't matter at Universal, where an army of underlings let not a comma go by without demanding a rewrite. And the novels, increasingly cerebral and unreal, seemed to have lost their compass. I was far away from completing Forster's vision of love fulfilled and unafraid to shout its name.

Gert never tried to steer me any differently. She didn't remotely understand how the movie business worked, beyond the adage that the writer was the lowest of the low in Hollywood. She gave me all the slack I needed, her fingers crossed that one of my antic scripts would get lucky and reach the screen. I was very full of myself in those years, fancying that I was developing a reputation as a wit, and that soon I would claim my place as a sort of latter-day Noel Coward, dry and effortless, skewering pretension.

It was somewhere in there that I visited Gert up at Sneden's, the trees on the river slope flaunting their gold in the sharp October light. We had birthdays just a week apart, and this was by way of a joint celebration: my thirty-two to her seventy-three. I think I was already starting to crack under the strain of my double career, with a half dozen scripts languishing on various desks of people with less and less power—

Hollywood's one-way ticket to Siberia. But I insisted to Gert that I was still in the game, determined to battle the odds till I produced a script as sublimely funny and sophisticated as *Private Lives*.

"But that was a play," Gert retorted mildly. And then she gave me a very Gert look, wry and penetrating, the ash of her upheld cigarette precariously long. "You know, he stood right where you're standing once," she said, and it took me half a beat to realize she meant Coward. "And he said, 'I don't know that I ever really had love in my life. Not the way I wanted it.'" Gert had been stunned, partly because she knew the two men who'd been Coward's longtime lovers, one and then the other, and they certainly had seemed to love *him*. Besides, Coward was the bard of romantic love: half the civilized world could whistle those songs of wistful longing for the perfect mate, "If Love Were All." Now it turned out that maybe even Noel Coward wasn't Noel Coward.

Within another year I'd hit the wall. I'd just finished writing a leaden script about vile people, called *The Hamptons*— suffice it to say that it paid the bills and made me feel like slime on dirty water. That summer my union decided to go on strike against the producers, demanding a cut of the video market. The six-month strike managed to derail all careers as marginal as mine, the kind that were based on fast talk and no screen credits. At the same time my editor in New York up and quit the company that had published my last four books. For the next three years I would try to peddle first one story and then another, on the strength of a hundred pages and an outline, only to find myself summarily rejected. Not hot anymore. By the end of that downward spiral I had a raft of rejection slips, enough to decoupage the walls of my study and then some.

My lowest point was the fall of '81, compounded by the end of a ruinous affair—two months' obsession and general self-destruction on my side, an enervated dalliance on his. And when it was over, I wouldn't let it go. It was as if my hands were frozen on the steering wheel, my foot slamming the gas pedal, as I relived again the self-abuse of falling in love with straight boys. The endless crash-and-burn of my adolescent crushes, all the way up to my twenty-fifth year, coming round full circle and leaving me pining for a hustler. I'd thought my love for Roger would protect me from the heart's careening, but it didn't, not that year.

I withheld the truth from him instead, figuring the least I could do was keep the pain to myself. But didn't succeed at that either, only managing to blame my ashen countenance and sudden bursts of sobbing on the dead-end of my work. I went back into therapy, three hours a week. I can't stomach rereading my journal of those months of suicidal emptiness. There's nothing further to learn from it—except perhaps the tenacity of shame, still able to sting twelve years later. Roger and I came out the other side more or less intact, though the useless pain and grief took months to deaden. It was in the middle of all of that I finally wrote a play.

I don't think I even told Gert about it till after the first draft was done. In the beginning it had more to do with the mire I was in with Joel, the object of my fixation. He was writing a play himself, about Jews-for-Jesus, without the slightest anxiety about what he might face in trying to get it produced. I decided his was the proper attitude—that I'd spent too much time being channeled and second-guessed by producers and well-meaning editors, till my work felt like everyone's business but mine. I would just begin: Act I, Scene I.

Mine was a stubbornly old-fashioned play, as it turned out, a drawing room comedy set twenty years in the past. Did anyone even *have* a drawing room anymore? It didn't deter me in the least, once I'd set my focus. I went back and forth to French's on Sunset, buying single copies of faded comedies from between the Wars, plays stuck in the genteel past that nobody bothered to revive. They had butlers and cooks and intrusive in-laws, in and out through the French windows, all fifth business to the leading lady and leading man. And always a tart-tongued best friend for the lady, whiskey on her breath, as well as a smooth-talking troublemaker who snaked his way into Eden and turned the central marriage upside down.

By the time I finished the first scene I was hooked, taking pleasure in the act of writing for the first time in years. How was I to know it wasn't permitted anymore to write a play with eight characters, this being the age of downsizing? Bare stage, two or three actors—that's what producers were looking for. I hadn't bothered to scope out the system at all: the nurturing of playwrights in the regional theaters, a close-knit troupe of itinerants where everyone knew everyone else. The one thing that hadn't changed since Gert's time was Hollywood as anathema, at best a necessary evil as long as you didn't make it a habit.

I finished the draft in about four months and began to work with a director friend who has since abandoned the boards to work in soaps (an easy half-million a year and you get to live in New York). *He* was old enough to remember the fox-collar glamour of Kit Cornell and Ina Claire and the Lunts. He saw what I was trying to do with a long-abandoned form, saw it better perhaps than I, and didn't let me get away with a wasted line. I worked another four months on revisions, tightening up and trimming the excess foliage, jettisoning one character (but careful to save his best lines and sprinkle them around among the others).

At last I was ready to show it to Gert. I dispatched a copy to Sneden's Landing, waiting two weeks before I followed it up with a call. I needn't have worried: she loved it. So much so that she'd already called up two or three of her ancient producer friends to ask if they were in the market. A little while later she had to go into the hospital for minor surgery, and to have her regular confrontation with her doctors over the volume of cigarettes and vodka she consumed. Her niece,

Merloyd, told me that Gert's copy of *Just the Summers* was the prominent item on her bedside table, in case she could pitch it to some old friend with moneybags who came by to visit.

The old producers shook their heads. Marvelous play, they admitted, but far too many speaking parts and set in a world that was simply forgotten. Gert remained undiscouraged, no more willing to give it up now than she was the Camels and the Stoli. In the end I didn't need her connections; I managed to draw a coterie of enthusiasts on my own, which led to a group of staged readings, the closest I ever came to being produced. Fifty folding chairs in a loft, but if you squinted you could almost believe you were in a theater, that the actors weren't reading from scripts but living every line.

It was years before it dawned on me that I'd written a play for an audience of one—and Miss Gertrude Macy was that one. Doubtless all of us writers are always out to please someone—Forster and his mother again—but Gert was something rarer than that. If I made it well enough to knock *her* socks off, then it would bear a seal of pedigree that went all the way back to the glistering streets of Broadway in its prime. Gert showed up at the loft on Ninth Avenue for the first reading, wearing her funeral duds, decades older than everyone else, and laughed her booming laugh at all the jokes she already knew. It was later that night that she took me and Roger to '21,' when I asked if it went too fast.

By the following autumn the play had a producer and a director and an improbable semi-commitment from Donald Sutherland to star. Thus we were suddenly locked into a Broadway production, raising our costs from the eighty thousand that would have sufficed for a ninety-nine seater to something over seven hundred thousand. It seemed an impossible gamble, but hard to resist. Our next reading was in a cavernous apartment in the Dakota, gargoyles peering in and a crowd of fat-cats in the folding chairs, possible investors. "You can smell the money," murmured Gert as she leaned toward me.

I was out at Sneden's a couple of evenings later, still flush from the performance at the Dakota, with how moving Sutherland had been as Julian, a man who'd chosen the closet in order to marry straight and rich. I remember Gert and I actually talking about individual theaters, which ones would work in the play's favor, and incidentally what great plays had trod the boards there previously. I was very high on the dream that night.

Around midnight we'd both stopped talking at last, a feat in itself, since the two of us could go on for hours. Gert was drinking her nightcap as we sat before the fire, while I puffed on a roach—a tableau worthy of a post-mod *Candida.* And when she quietly asked about this "gay cancer" she'd been reading about, I realized it had been on her mind all evening. This must have been the winter of '83, before César or anyone else I knew had fallen. So far it was all just shadowy rumors, an East Coast thing, I retorted with a careless laugh, assuring her it had nothing to do with Roger and me. The pinnacle of my earliest denial.

And I remember it didn't appease her, the worried crease only seeming to deepen in the firelight. But we let it go for the moment, for the sake of the circle of security we provided for one another. Only when I was leaving, as she dropped me off at the bridge to get a taxi, did she squeeze my hand and say, "Be careful."

There was one other time, a few months later. I was back and forth to New York quite a bit that year, having been hired to write a script about a model who becomes the billboard face of the moment. *15 Minutes,* it was called, and I cared about it a lot because it had an up-front gay character who was the heroine's best friend and roommate. I barely had time to talk to Gert on the phone, but managed to hold an evening open before my return to L.A. There was snow on the ground at Sneden's, a late winter that stubbornly wouldn't yield to spring.

I can't say Gert was in somber spirits, or any less ebullient to have me for an evening to herself. Curious, but she never seemed to age during that decade I knew her—never aged *further,* I mean, than the beautiful wrinkled terrain of the face I saw the day I met her. I would have said that night that she was the same as ever, indomitable; but then I was the one who could still laugh off the darkness about to engulf us all.

"I have to go into the hospital again," she said with a certain breeziness. "They think there's a spot on my lung." She was puffing a cigarette even as she said it.

Then *I* was the one who got gloomy. Could it be cancer? Yes, of course. But they could treat it, right? They were catching it early, right? She shrugged, somehow not all that concerned. She'd always hoped to reach eighty, she said, but after that she knew it was a free-fall. And then she started to reminisce about the ones she'd lost to cancer, and here the passion surfaced. First her beloved younger sister, then Kit—both had died in the age of discretion, when genteel people thought it best not to tell the truth to the dying. "Oh, it was terrible. They got sicker and sicker, and we'd all put on our brave faces and tell them they were going to be *fine.*" She fired that last word with fierce regret.

And what did she think death was? I asked her. Nothing, she replied, matter-of-fact. But what about the white light and the tunnel? I persisted. Lately there had been much to-do among those who studied near-death experiences, people who'd gone to the brink and back, the welcoming committee of loved ones beckoning them into the light. No, said Gert, she gave that no credence at all: "That's just the brain shutting down." There was something heroic about her lack of sentimentality, consistent with her belief that when it was time to go you made your own choice and pressed your own button. No extraordinary measures to keep the body pumping. I remember hoping I'd be that way myself when it got to be closer to my time—but that was forty years away, long enough to get used to death.

Merloyd writes to me that Gert's stoicism in the face of illness and death didn't mean she wasn't a believer in her own way:

> *She would tell me in the last years of her life that at certain moments she would feel a kind of euphoria. She felt that perhaps it was what came to people who meditate. She somehow knew intuitively how to step outside of time. The very way she chose to live, facing the river, facing the sea, rescuing stray dogs and sticking by old friends and wayward family when anyone else's last shred of tolerance would have snapped, was a kind of celebration, even worship of life.*

I didn't hear from Gert all that summer, but didn't worry, assuming I would have heard if anything was wrong—forgetting that proud instinct of hers, discretion at all costs and never a bother to anyone. When I thought of Gert I pictured her at the Vineyard, still clocking noon by mixing herself a bullshot, stuffed avocados as usual on the deck. Indeed she was, says Merloyd, in a turban to mask the effects of the chemo. I don't even remember what my deadline was that summer, or whether Donald Sutherland had pulled out by then, or if the producer had already washed his hands of the whole thing. In any case my poor play was moribund and orphaned, and I hated to think of telling Gert, who had been so much its champion.

October came, and our birthdays. Because I couldn't rouse her on the phone, I sent flowers to Sneden's Landing. The card read: "Happy 79 from Happy 38." Roger and I were busily getting ready for an autumn trip to Tuscany, so I didn't think to follow up on the roses. But a couple of days later the florist called to say they couldn't deliver the order. Why not?

"The lady's in the hospital, sir." Well then, I answered briskly, have them delivered there. A day later the stakes escalated. The florist again, apologizing because they couldn't deliver them to the hospital either. I knew and I didn't know. I placed a call to the hospital and was told I should "talk to the family," the first time I'd ever heard that particular sidestep. The euphemisms of dying hadn't flooded my vocabulary yet.

I spoke with Merloyd, fumbling a condolence, hardly conscious yet of what I'd just lost. The family was planning a memorial lunch at Sneden's, but Roger and I had to decline because we'd be in Italy on that day. I lit a candle for Gert in Florence, in Brunelleschi's soaring gray-stone church of Santo Spirito, a believer in beauty if nothing else. Returning from that trip, Roger and I were seized by the emergency of César's diagnosis, and on and on till all of our friends were consumed one way or another, dying themselves or taking care of the stricken.

I hadn't much time for reflection once the plague had taken root. When I'd think of Gert it was always bittersweet— a word Coward practically invented—recalling a vanished world before the war. Our war. I understand now that it wasn't just a friend who'd been taken from me, but an elder and a mentor. Gert was my pioneer, a link to the dreams that made me different, the push I needed to go my own way. I don't think I ever thanked her in so many words, but following her lead I refuse to regret that. No regrets.

Of course, no one knows who *The Barretts* are anymore, or Kit or Coward or the Lunts. It won't be long, I suppose, before we come to a place where even Garbo and Dietrich will draw a blank. All of them are just a sidelight, anyway, to the history of the gay and lesbian struggle. Glamorous though the closet was, the world Gert and her friends inhabited still had walls, so that they didn't even think to reach out to the pained anonymous legions of queers with nobody to look up to. Maybe history wasn't ready yet. In any case, I can't bring myself to condemn them for their silence and their compromise. It needed a revolution to challenge us all, a moment after which there would be no going back: Stonewall.

I don't know if Gert reached out to me, or I to her. It was doubtless mutual. In my play there's a character called Robin, a balmy old woman poet in a wheelchair who lived in Paris in the twenties and knew them all. She keeps calling the young man in the play Ernest, mistaking him for Hemingway. Robin isn't quite Gert, who never suffered a moment's lapse of clarity, but the same historical linkage was there. And at the end of the play, when the young man, Tom, has broken with Julian and is off on his own to Paris, he has one last question for his mentor. "Does it go too fast?" he asks.

"You mean life?" retorts Julian. "Just the summers."

Gert proved wrong in the end. It *has* gone too fast, so swift and sudden I sometimes feel I've been left clutching the empty air as life rocketed by. Gert swore I wouldn't feel at the end that I hadn't had enough, but then she couldn't know the seismic convulsion that AIDS would unleash. Frankly, I'm glad she didn't live to see the decimation of the arts, by plague and then by Philistines. Better for her to sit on the bluff of her memories, cheerfully giving it all away to me, though never stuck in the past herself. My friend from the far country of the eighth decade, first among sisters. Providing me my most intense experience of age, a cider taste of a world I would never reach myself except through her. All that and the Broadway years besides, *my* Broadway years. Caviar extra, but who can quibble with such a banquet? Or two on the aisle in Row H, as a thousand curtains rise.

MY PRIESTS

I DIDN'T IN FACT RECALL his first letter, or the phone call that followed it up. My number was still listed then, so it must have been the summer of '89, before the death threats and the bricks through my windows. Apparently he asked if we could meet, for he had just relocated here from back east, to become the associate pastor at Saint Anselm's in West Hollywood. I wasn't unintrigued, having heard rumors for years that the bilious Inquisitor who ran Saint Anselm's was notorious for denying funeral Masses to gay Catholics who'd died of AIDS. The new priest, Father Gambone, would doubtless defend his superior and dismiss these ugly tales as just more Catholic-bashing. In any case I was too busy, too swamped by Stephen's illness, to spare a cup of coffee. Call me back in a few months, I told Gambone, and perhaps we could snatch an hour together.

But I warn you, I added playfully, *I'll want to know all the dirt on how many priests are gay.*

He never called back; I never gave it another thought. Well, once or twice. I'd turn off Sunset at Tower Records, craning to find a parking space, cursing the long swath of yellow curb in front of Saint Anselm's, the empty parking lot beside the parish house. And I'd wonder about that young priest—from Philadelphia, wasn't he?—and whether he'd made a dent in the bigotry and the Roman lies about our people. A year or so later, when that bloodsucker convent opened just outside the walls of Auschwitz, defiling every murdered Jew with its simpering Carmelite prayers—I remember thinking in the midst of the flap how very like Saint Anselm's was this particular Polish insult. Saint Anselm's, perched with its pretty shrubbery and its knelling tower on the very lip of the cauldron of AIDS. As if the very thing West Hollywood needed for its hobbled tribe, here in the first gay city in America, was a Catholic presence on the hill.

But this is to give the one little church on Holloway Drive far more importance than it deserved. My fight was with the Axis powers in Rome, the Vatican Nazis. My various fulminations on the subject had engendered a fair amount of response, especially from recovering Catholics, whose white-hot rage and sense of violation by the Church made my own anger seem puny by comparison.

I'd also been in contact with several priests and sisters, fearless ones who chose to fight within the system, as well as a lot of ex-religious. I couldn't be said to have mellowed exactly, always ready to flash a moon, rhetorically speaking, at the Polish Pope and his diabolical sidekick, Cardinal Ratzinger, the Vatican's Minister of Hate. But I had also come to see how passionate and self-denying were the good men and women still in uniform—feminist nuns who dared to be pro-choice; the radical left and its Liberation Theology, fighting the generals in Latin America; the Catholic Workers and the underclass, not a money-changer among them. I had begun to appreciate, in other words, the commitment the best of them had to service, especially to serving their gay and lesbian brethren. Thus did I cheer the defiance of Dignity, who refused to be ignored or tossed out or barred from the sacraments just because their love didn't fit the psychopathology of church dogma.

Then, midsummer this year, came the you-may-not-remember-me letter. Father Gambone! He began by apologizing for his silence, but admitted I'd scared him off with my rant against Rome in various interviews. He felt "unjustly condemned," he said, having given over his ministry for ten years to serving people with AIDS. The rest of him secretly agreed with the things I said, but he couldn't face that and go on with his work. As it turned out, he didn't need me anyway. Early on in Gambone's tenure at Saint Anselm's, a young professor named Joseph was serving ten o'clock Mass with the priest. They caught one another's eye and fell in love, just like that. A moment of transubstantiation if there ever was one.

He didn't say how much time they had for sheer joy before the darkness fell. Only now did I understand that Gambone was fifty-five, and had been out for fifteen years to his family, his Jesuit order, indeed the Church. I don't know why he didn't get the boot for being so honest, probably because he kept his vow of chastity. Even with Joseph. And then like a sick joke, still on the honeymoon, the young teacher fell ill. The soul-crushing torture of AIDS took over. Gambone spared me the details, and tried after burying Joseph to pour his grief into deeper commitment. Hard to say if it worked, or how disconcerting it must've been for the flock, watching the priest break down sobbing in the middle of Mass.

Now I want to share some things with you. I'm moving back to Philadelphia, leaving the Jesuits, the priesthood and the Church, as the final stage of my coming out. It was a half-truth that by staying in I could be more effective because wearing the collar opened the trust lines faster and deeper than without it. What finally made me see the essential dishonesty of my rationalizations was the latest assault from the Vatican supporting discrimination against us in several basic

*areas of civil rights (in effect wanting us dead) and suggesting
that the American bishops extend this homophobic influence
to America at large, "to promote the public morality of the
entire civil society on the basis of fundamental moral values."*

*That did it. There was no ambiguity here—just raw preju-
dice, hyperhomophobia, ignorance, cloaked in sanctimonious
pietism. I swallowed hard when past utterances came forth,
from Ratzinger, kicking my friend John McNeil out of the
Order, etc. etc. Shame on me! This latest pogrom finally put
it all into focus, and now I don't see how I could have stayed
as long as I have.*

Still a long-winded Jesuit, collar or no. I tried to reach
him, but he'd already left for Philly. A brave man, and clearly
one after my own heart. Imagine, starting life over after forty
years in the order and twenty-five as a priest. But what really
tugged at me was how the Church had gotten off so easily—
just another resignation, a failure of one man's calling. How
far up the hierarchy did anyone know about Joseph, or the
love that finally made Gambone human? They only knew
about one kind of gay priest anyway, the kind that diddled
altar boys.

The tortured secret life of the pedophile, and all the
Church's power mustered to keep things hushed, no treatment
except a rest cure at a sylvan retreat. Then the transfer into a
new parish, the slate wiped clean until the diddling starts again.
The mess won't go away, of course. Stories have surfaced suggesting that the Church has shelled out three hundred million
dollars of late to settle the increasingly aggressive lawsuits
around the issue of sexual abuse. Not a good year for "suffer
the little children," what with the banner headlines about the
perv from Boston who got into the pants of dozens of kids
over a period of thirty years. Bless me, Father, for you have
sinned.

No idea, not a clue about what a healthy gay and lesbian relationship looks like. My friend Father Bernard tells me that most of the abusers aren't really pedophiles at heart. Rather, they're closeted men who took the vow of purity at twenty, determined to keep their baser instincts under control. A couple of decades of that neurotic self-denial, and then they hit a midlife crisis, and suddenly their dicks are driving them out of their minds. The altar boys and the CCD girls just happen to be the nearest warm bodies, the perfect obedient victims, stunned into silence by their veneration of the criminal.

Which brings us to the sick document perpetrated this summer, a Ratzinger special, the last straw for Father Gambone. It commands the bishops to fight against all legislation that mandates gay and lesbian rights of any sort, but especially the right to have children, natural or foster. And of course to keep such deviants away from schools or daycare centers, whatever might trigger the sin so common among the priesthood.

What would Jerry have made of it all, I wonder. Jerry Silver was the first ex-monk I ever knew—a Trappist for years, on a farm in Ohio, keeping bees and boiling up the harvest fruit for jam. By the time I met him in '78, he'd been out of the order for more than a decade, but still looked rather like a road-company Friar Tuck, portly and jolly and a little mad. He'd taken the name Jerry Silver upon reentering civilian life because he wanted to express solidarity with his Jewish friends. Not that he had such dark memories of the cloistered life. "I loved being a monk," he'd say. "The hot lunch program was fabulous. And every Easter we'd all go over to Rome for the parties. I always stuck with the Kennedys, because they got invited *everywhere*."

So how many priests and monks are gay? I'd ask, to needle him. What did he think the percentages were? He'd flutter his pudgy hands, spotted with the scars of bee stings and covered with rings like a gypsy. "Oh my dear, who can say? A hundred and ten percent. No wonder it took me so long to decide—I really wanted to be a *nun,* not a priest."

And so he was on special occasions—Halloween without fail, but any good party would do. He had a closetful of habits, from billowing tents and wimples of the days before Vatican II to pert little modified numbers. He'd acquired them from an obscure specialty shop downtown, a sort of nuns' department store, ingratiating himself with the staff by telling them he was buying for his sister, cloistered somewhere in the wilderness. "But do you know her size?" they fretted. "Oh, she's a big girl," Jerry retorted. "Just about my size."

I remember vividly the New Year's brunch at Jerry's place in Mount Washington. He was dressed in full Mother Superior drag, flouncing about in Seventh Heaven. The cross that swung from his neck was hauntingly beautiful, hammered bronze, ancient without a doubt. The heft of it in your hand was like a stone. "This old thing?" said Jerry, showing it off. "I picked it up at the Vatican. Coptic, I think. Ninth century, somebody told me once."

Picked it up how, exactly? Suddenly Jerry's face went rosy pink in his wimple, but he couldn't resist the story either. It seems that every year when the Trappists made their Roman pilgrimage, they signed up for a private tour of the Vatican treasuries. A wizened keeper of the keys—an old, half-blind padre with skin the texture of tissue paper—would lead them through banks of embroidered vestments, altar linens so fine they would've melted in your mouth. On to the gem-encrusted chalices, the Mannerist candelabras as tall as a man, the icons, the reliquaries. It was an Aladdin's cave of booty and plunder, the raw material of power, so much that even the Vatican didn't have enough end tables to display it. Byzantium crushed and pagan Rome, a thousand infidels' temples looted, all for the sake of a secret trove. One imagined the Pope taking a bath in his gold like Scrooge McDuck in his vault.

"To us," shrugged Jerry, "it was like a white sale at

Bloomingdale's. We'd grab up a handful of linen and stuff it into our cassocks. Maybe a nice gold salver or an incense-burner. The old queen never noticed. This cross was just hanging from a *nail*. I figured if I didn't snatch it, then somebody else would. Some pious Dominican, probably."

For a moment I was open-mouthed with shock, imagining an imminent lightning bolt or a Vatican goon squad storming the door. How many years must you spend in Purgatory for burgling the Vatican? Of course I understood that most of the stuff was stolen in the first place, or at least bled from the faithful poor. Whatever you said about Jerry's blasphemy, you couldn't accuse him of being a hypocrite.

I thought of Chaucer, and his gaggle of pilgrims making their way to Canterbury. Six hundred years ago the poet had the clergy's number: the Pardoner selling his indulgences, heaven on the lay-away plan; the sensuous Prioress shivering as she eats her oysters, relishing the tale she tells of a boy murdered by Jews; the Friar and the Summoner, snarling with contempt as they cast each other as the villain of their opposing fables. Bring that crew to the Vatican treasury for a little Easter tour, and the stealing would be so brazen they'd be clanking like knights in armor by the time they came out the other side.

"If gold can rust," Chaucer observes, clucking his tongue over all that ecclesiastical corruption, "then what will iron do?" Jerry Silver didn't fret for a moment about such niceties of ethics. What he'd taken from his years in the Church was a feel for camp, the ridiculous self-importance of the queens in power. In any case Jerry had other reasons for leaving the order, the gay and lesbian revolution first among them. He moved directly from the monastery into a gay commune in L.A. His natural role was to mother the rest of them, meanwhile keeping the commune in jam and honey, cupboards full. And yet what he really longed for was a man to love him back.

He was hopelessly naive, though, as to how to go about

it. He'd fall discreetly for one or another of the beautiful and damned young men of Hollywood. But *so* discreet was his courting dance that the young men never picked up on it, even if they'd wanted to respond—which they probably wouldn't have, given Jerry's vast self-deprecation, the shyness about his rotund shape and his vanishing hair. But he always maintained a brave smile and a deep-throated laugh, with no self-pity that I ever saw. He had a certain simple faith that things were going to turn out all right—even after his two partners in the nursing service he'd founded embezzled the business out from under him, leaving him penniless.

With his pride and his grin still intact, he set off for Europe. This was just before the plague hit full-force in L.A. No question but that Jerry would've made a fortune with his registry nurses, one of those boom businesses that got rich off AIDS. But Jerry was never one to maunder over spilled milk, and within two years he'd set himself up as curator for a huge modernist art collection in Paris. He lived in a shoebox of an apartment, and most important, found himself a boyfriend in Amsterdam. Sporadically, one or the other of us would pick up the phone in the middle of the night to check in, never getting the time lag right.

"I've got everything I want," he'd say. "I always knew my European years would be my triumph." And where was the Coptic cross? I asked him. "On a nail right beside my bed," he laughed.

We fell out of touch during Roger's illness, and by the time Roger died, the young Dutchman was sick. We were a pair of widows when Jerry and I spoke again. I could hear the rattle in his voice, the struggle to breathe, and knew he would be next. But he'd managed to finish the five-pound catalogue of the art collection, and shepherded the paintings to Washington for a triumphant exhibition at the Smithsonian, collapsing with pneumocystis as soon as he returned to Paris.

"Don't worry about me. I've had everything I ever

wanted," he declared defiantly. Not a twinge of regret, or any self-consciousness about speaking in the past tense. "I only have one more thing on my list. I *have* to go first class on the QE2 before I die. I'll sell the damn cross if I have to."

But AIDS caught up with him first, leaving his life list unfinished. It was weeks after he died that one of his old friends in L.A. called me with the news. I gathered he went surrounded by his Paris friends, bohemians of the old style who filled his room with art talk. He died without a *sou*, I was given to understand. I didn't protest about the Coptic cross, having no claim on it myself. But I rather hoped one of his bedside vigilants was a medievalist, with the wit to slip it off the nail and pocket it. Jerry would've appreciated such a transfer—anything to keep it from those Dominicans.

Father Gambone and Brother Jerry. Is either of these a story with a happy ending? Not that it's for me to judge, but I can't help thinking there was sufficient joy and recovered self-esteem for both in the mere act of leaving the Church. Two more sprung from the savage ignorance and soul-destroying dogma, the two thousand years of belittling women, the enslavement of overpopulation. Every abandonment of vocation strikes a blow against the long history of evil perpetrated by the powers of Rome.

And yet it gives me scant comfort these days to see how the Church flails, more and more erratically, to pretend its history never happened. For history is its collaborator down the centuries, somehow never connecting the dots between the blood-soaked past and the outrages of the present. The Inquisition's reign of terror in Europe, burning at the stake anyone who stood up to their hypocrisy, indeed anyone who looked at them funny; the systematic wiping out of the pagan texts after Constantine converted to Christianity in 313. You must destroy the documents if you mean to rewrite history, leaving your own version of events as the only truth. Or take the lunatic presumptions of the Syllabus of Errors, Pope Pius

IX's catalogue of heresies issued in 1864. A veritable paean to ignorance, condemning religious liberty, all liberty for that matter; against science, against progress, against the separation of church and state; establishing control over all literature, over public education. And how does history report all this? On bended knee, of course, because it won't do to be condemning religion. After all, the Vatican *means* well, doesn't it?

No, it doesn't. Centuries of oppression have been papered over with quaintness, with a picturesque sentimentality as prettily inoffensive as a line of girls in First Communion whites. I'm glad I lived long enough to see a pop star rip up the Pope's picture on national television, even if it has meant enduring the prissy backlash. Either you speak nicely about this "holy man," or you button your lip. In just this way the eyes of history avert their gaze from the collaboration of Pius XII and the Nazis. A real piece of work, old number XII, who wouldn't intervene even so far as to tell his Polish cardinals to dampen the enthusiasm of the good Catholics running the camps and the ovens. And this at a time when the war was virtually over, the Allied victory assured. You just wash your hands of the final wave of victims—and anyway, how many tears does a Pope really need to shed over the settling of that ancient score, those Jews who killed Our Lord?

It was fascinating recently to watch the Church rewrite its history again, and this time in public. As if it were actual news, His Holiness accepted the findings of a thirteen-year commission and officially withdrew the charges of heresy against Galileo. All with an utterly straight face, and reported by the press with a big dose of cuddly quaintness—a harmless ritual, wave to Papa. No feel for the degrading of scientific truth, the personal horror of Galileo's reluctant recantation, because he'd proven that the universe wasn't earth-centered at all. Galileo died broken, his last eight years under house arrest in Siena, while all the Church ignoramuses and black-cowled torturers went scot-free. And now, three hundred and sixty years later,

the Polish Pope merely accuses them of "imprudent opposi-
tion"—a bare, limp-wristed sissy's slap.

So apparently all we have to do, we gay and lesbian here-
tics, is wait a few hundred years, and the bubble-enclosed Pope
of 2350 will swish his skirts and declare it's all been a misun-
derstanding. Don't hold your breath, kids. The Copernican
theory of cosmic motion is one thing, sexuality quite another.
The latter is only for making babies, starving ones ideally, because they make better copy and bring in more gold to Rome.
Pleasure is forbidden, intimacy more so. Your deepest secrets
belong to the Church as well, waiting behind the grille of the
confessional. How many gay Catholics have told me of being
forced by an overeager priest to tell more and more lurid details of a harmless jerkoff session?

Obviously I haven't been in the market for rapprochement
with Rome. When I had the first letters from priests, after
Borrowed Time was published, they were quick to apologize for
the excesses of Cardinal Ratzinger and his Boss. This was a
terrible time, they agreed—a return to the Dark Ages of intolerance—but the only way to face it was to take the long view.
The Polish Pope wouldn't be forever. He hadn't yet utterly
broken the spirit of renewal that seemed a kind of miracle to
the participants of Vatican II. Pray for another John XXIII.
The new Inquisition would pass. Meanwhile, of course, they
were praying for me, if that was all right.

Except it wasn't all right, and gave me the creeps besides.
I replied that their awesome patience and hope for a better age
was of no use to gay and lesbian people who were being wiped
out by our own holocaust. And if it wasn't the same as Europe's holocaust, with as many as eleven million "innocent"
dead, the response of the Church was exactly the same—the
washing of hands in the same bowl of dirty water, slick with
the scum of piety. Don't pray for me, please, I declared. Start
the revolution instead.

But the letters trickled in anyway, and I couldn't ignore the passion with which they spoke about their work fighting AIDS. AIDS, they said, was where Jesus would be. AIDS was the place where they would learn the transforming power of love. Sounded good, but I was still suspicious of their motives; it was as if they were chalking up points for sainthood. I wasn't quite so far gone in cynicism as my friend Pat, whose flame-red Italian opinion was that the only thing Mother Teresa ever aspired to in her life was to be on the cover of *People*. I understood the sentiment, but really there were limits. Yet recently I've come to hear rumors that she won't permit the lovers of gay people with AIDS to visit their dying partners in her hospices. Only the family, please. And her Missionary Sisters of Charity—or so it has filtered through the underground—withhold pain medication from patients, asking them to offer their pain to God.

I think the first crack in my own cynicism was Brother Toby. A publisher sent me the manuscript of *Morning Glory Babies,* Toby's account of a lay Catholic community in rural northern California, where he lived with Sister Marti and Sister Julie. They were taking in babies with AIDS, otherwise abandoned, and lovingly caring for them. What was so moving and humbling about the story was its plain-spoken joy, genuine in ways a hypocrite couldn't fake. They kept themselves solvent by running a Christmas tree farm on their land near Santa Rosa. Of course all the babies died eventually, guttering like so many candles, but in the meantime there were birthdays and holidays, a farmhouse rippling with laughter.

I still don't know if Toby and Marti and Julie belong to any official order, but I rather think not. They don't appear to owe any special fealty to Rome, defining their mission by the largeness of their hearts. Not a scrap of brocade in sight. Now I order a tree every year from Starcross, and Sister Julie scrawls a note on the packing crate to wish me well. Toby and I

maintain an off-and-on correspondence, for he has enthusiastically read all my books, no matter how anti-Church they
are. He has, as I've come to learn, bigger things to worry
about.

When he read in the news about the hospital wards of
children in Romania, tainted by AIDS-infected blood and
chained to their cribs as they stared hollowly at the ceiling,
Toby flew over to see what he could do. There was a haunting
scrap of footage on "PrimeTime Live," where he scooped up
one of the babies and carried him outside into a ruined garden.
A child who had never played or laughed, probably never been
out of the crib—and his face was suffused with delight, just to
be held and to see the sun in the trees.

I remember thinking Toby was taking on too much, that
he couldn't take care of *every* AIDS baby, certainly not a whole
country's worth. But he has persevered, and the Starcross
newsletter reports every quarter on their progress, teaching ignorant nurses how to care, tearing down the prison walls. You
cannot help but transpose it against the dark little item that
landed Starcross in the local papers in Santa Rosa. One night
they had an emergency, one of the kids had stopped breathing,
and they called the volunteer fire department for help, to bring
the kid to the nearest emergency room. And the firemen
wouldn't come, because they might catch it.

One thing I've learned from this unspeakable age of suffering is how myriad are the ways to lash out against the darkness.
Enormous though the power is in the hate councils of the
Vatican, there's still room for a little saintliness far off the
beaten track, at a complete remove from the hierarchs and
patriarchs. Perhaps I've even come to oversentimentalize the
God-work of Toby and the sisters—the atheist's sin, to get
maudlin in the end, and over things you'd never get away with
in a novel, like those Christmas trees.

You grow attached to goodness when you know it's the
real thing. Still, it's a bit unnerving to be the recipient of a

holy card, an icon of Mother and Child that fell from the folds of Toby's letter about a week ago.

> *I will play surrogate to one of your nun great-aunts and send this to you—the traditional Catholic answer to every problem. This one is put out by a Catholic AIDS group. They are one of the less "brocaded" parts of my troubled church. When they began there was a lot of posturing for who would be the boss AIDS priest, but the epidemic has purified them. The epidemic has purified us all.*

"Your brother, Toby," it was signed, and I saw it was the plain truth; we were a brotherhood of warriors. I didn't even flinch that Toby's God was in there somewhere. At least it wasn't the Pope's God.

About two years ago I began to correspond with Father Tom, a priest from an order I'd never heard of, chaplain to a college way out in Idaho. He enthusiastically endorsed my brickbats against the Vatican, then told me about his own AIDS work. It sounded as if he knew every case in the state personally—barely a dozen when he arrived, but no support systems in place, all kept secret and isolated like a shuttered cabin on the Great Divide. Tom found that though there was no visible gay and lesbian community in Idaho, there was at least an unspoken network. He moved through it to find the sick, comforting them and drawing them together to help one another.

We've met several times, Father Tom and I, and he's never once mentioned the name of God. If what he's doing out there in Idaho is spreading the Gospel, he doesn't put it to me in those terms. We talk about the *politics* of God, and especially about the witch hunt being engineered in Rome against our people. He leans toward the sixty percent figure when considering our numbers in the clergy. He has successfully come out to most of the powers of his order, who only warn him not to be too public. No one can call him a sinner, because he's chaste—technically speaking.

And I find myself rooting for him, not even impatient that he doesn't publicly spit in the Church's face, for he's part of the underground instead, a leader in the Resistance. This means he runs retreats in which gay and lesbian issues are out on the table. He works his own network of queer clergy, offering his counsel to the fearfully closeted. On the clerical grapevine, he hears of more than a couple of bishops with live-in lovers. Rumors frustrating to Tom, for these pointy-hats take no public stance against the Church. Hey, I've got mine, Jack, leave me alone.

Tom plans to study in Rome next year, beating the scholar/dictators at their own game, ferreting out all the loopholes in the Paulist gibberish about the separation of sex and love. Meanwhile he's got his priorities straight—or *not* straight, I should say. Two months ago I asked him over dinner in a queer restaurant—his eyes darting about with delight, drawn by so much merriment among his brothers and sisters— I asked him what would happen if he met a man the way Gambone had. Someone to love. And Tom looked at me, a frown of intensity creasing his cherub's face, and snapped his fingers. "I'd be out of the priesthood like that," he said.

To me that's not hypocrisy, but a man keeping open the options of the heart; options Tom and I agree were not available to previous generations of priests—or so they thought, cowed more by their own self-hatred than by the dogma. It's the same pattern we see in the current Jeremiah generation of homophobes, that priss tribe of right-wing pundits and op-ed loonies, the Pentecostal preachers coifed like Liberace, mincing and fluttering as they harangue us wayward Sodomites. Never a breath about gay women, for to them it's a fight to the death between one kind of man and another. They've got a white-knuckle grip on heterosex themselves, a decision they made in their youth to escape their own carnal ambiguity, the guilt of their secret desires.

And they're welcome to it, that desperate choice of straightness, or in the priests' case, celibacy. But what they cannot bear about *us* in the post-Stonewall world is how alive we are with pride, how connected to one another. We are laying to rest the shame and self-recrimination, and they're frantic to shut us up. We reflect too bright a mirror back on them. Meanwhile the old priest, sitting alone in his kitchen, sloshed on communion wine, shakes his head with bitter rue because the world has passed him by. To him it's not fair that his younger brethren live out their gayness openly, going so far as to think of it as one of the gifts of the Spirit. They ought to be *suffering* their sexuality, the way he has, or what's the point?

As a non-believer I speak, of course, as a rank outsider. I have no sense of the God side in all of this, except what people tell me. Perhaps I protest too much that none of it touches me. I sometimes think I've ended up an atheist who's still an Episcopalian at heart, glad to share community with the fighter-priests, no matter if I think the founding story is just a pretty myth. And yet there have been occasions that have spoken to me in words of another tongue, an aligning of my pagan faith in the goddess of love and the god of the sun with a larger sense of connectedness, a mystery without politics.

In the late spring before Stephen died, we went on a cruise of the Greek islands and the coast of Asia Minor. Our ship a tub that stunk like rancid cooking oil, rust raining down from the joints whenever we hit a swell. Eight hundred passengers, who mostly came to buy tee-shirts and carpets and usually skipped the ruins. By the time we landed at Dikili in southern Turkey, to make the trek inland to ancient Ephesus, most of our fellow travelers opted to stay on deck and broil their sullen midwestern flesh. The bus was only a third full as we set off through the dusty hills. Melek, our tour guide in knockoff Chanel, explained to us that the sea had receded six miles since the glory days of the port of Ephesus. Now it lay stranded in the desert, a white ghost marble city.

The winding road through those six miles was mostly moonscape, too salty to be arable, only the low hills that must have once been islands bearing a choke of chaparral and a scatter of date palms. Melek ordered the driver to pull over, stopping us in the middle of nowhere. Stevie and I peered anxiously out, wondering if a terrorist attack was on the program. "See over there in the field," said Melek, pointing across the arid scrub. "See that column?"

You had to adjust to the waves of shimmering heat, more blinding than any Ray Bans could shade. But now that she mentioned it, there *was* a column out there, with a nest of cranes at the top. It was, she told us, the last column of the Temple of Diana—one of the Seven Wonders of the ancient world—at least the last column that was still in place. All the rest had been hauled off to Istanbul to ring the inner dome of Hagia Sophia, one religion erasing another. The dark green marble pillar in the field was improbable and forlorn, but from it had flowed, like ripples in a pond, a whole world of pagan temples, crowning every promontory.

Then Melek told us to shift our gaze about thirty degrees to the right, where the rubble of a Venetian fort sprawled across a rise. A village was clustered beneath its walls, abandoned it looked like to us, unless they were all in there napping, fleeing the heat of the day. A tiny barrel church anchored the houses at one end—Orthodox, Coptic, I couldn't have said. "Now, do you see the house just below the church?" she asked us. We nodded. More like a sway-roofed stable, really. "In that house Saint John finished writing the Gospel."

She spoke without any melodrama, a Muslim herself, though clearly no mullah was going to make her shed her Chanel, real or otherwise. To her this was a purely secular experience, with no more symbolic weight to the pagan land-mark than to the Christian. Myself, I couldn't stop staring, for here we were at a *writer's* landmark. Factoids came back from my confirmation classes in the fifties. John's Gospel—the beautiful one, the record of a poet—written some eighty years after the events it records. And on this hill he had formed the final awestruck sentence—in Greek, on a parchment scroll:

And there are also many other things which Jesus did. If they should be written every one, I suppose that even the world itself could not contain the books that should be written.

We couldn't have been there more than two minutes alto-gether, and the choking bus was already revving up for the twisted climb to Ephesus. This had all been just a sidelight. Yet I yearned to stay longer, to sprint across the salt fields and run my hand down the pocked marble; then to lope up the rise to John's house, to peer in and try to imagine him work-ing. I pictured him like Saint Jerome in his study in Dürer's great engraving, only without the lion.

Was this a religious experience? Well, not the conven-tional kind. Indeed, it was two religions—the pagan, face to face with the Christian, mute testimony to the schism of two worlds, before and after. Fragments and echoes, more like phantoms than physical places now, no signs or roadside mark-ers to point the way. When Melek is running late, doubtless she skips this two-minute stop entirely. As we pulled away I craned for a last look. What quickened my spirit was the oppo-sition of these two memories, pagan and Christian. You couldn't say from the evidence here which would prevail in the end. No priest, no exegesis would settle the matter. The deep past is just a pillar in a field and a sagging barn.

Or go back to the fall of '87, when my friend Craig and I wandered for ten days in Italy. He wasn't even as sick as I am now—didn't die till New Year's of '91—but we both believed this Tuscan journey would be his final voyage out. In all the years I'd known him he'd never had a buck to spare, writing as he did for the gay press, which more or less paid him in rice and beans. I had two free tickets from a mileage club and offered him the world for his birthday, wherever he'd like to go. "Florence," he answered instantly, as if he'd been waiting all his life to be asked.

Not an easy trip for me, who'd spent a glorious week with Roger there in '83. Too soon. But off we trekked—and found ourselves in a fusty *pensione* six floors up and facing the Arno, the Ponte Vecchio just below and a vista across the roofs of the city, that brandy light of mid-November. *Perfecto,* most especially the two spinster proprietresses who appeared to have sprung full-blown out of *A Room with a View*. Yet these two estimable ladies would always squabble at the comparison. Oh no, they assured us, Forster was three blocks up the street, at Signore Rotelli's. Not a first-class establishment, clearly, round the bend and out of sight of the Old Bridge. Now Mrs. *Browning's* view was quite superb, just two doors down, a lovely place to die.

A lovely place to die became our mantra for the rest of that trip—standing on the terrace at San Miniato, or the piazza of the Virgin's Cloak in Siena, or the top of a cracked tower in San Gimignano. And yet it turned out that Craig had been seriously misinformed about where you had to go to see the masterworks of Tuscany. After ten minutes' shivering impatience in the Duomo, he categorically refused to go into another church, so bitter was he about the Vatican's edicts of hate against our tribe. Wouldn't go back in to see the Giottos, or the Fra Angelico *Annunciation* in the stairhall at San Marco. He was only interested in the secular, the *David* most especially, and had to restrain himself from spitting when flocks of nuns went skittering by with their guidebooks.

Trumped therefore by an anti-Popery deeper even than

mine, I was forced to revisit alone the holy places I had come
to love before. In practice this amounted to trailing around
from one Brunelleschi building to another, especially the soaring interior of Santo Spirito and the jewel-box perfection of
the Pazzi Chapel. And yet they did nothing for me this time,
less than nothing really, the unbearable serenity just another
goad to my grief and solitude. I had somehow talked myself
out of the one peaceable compromise I'd made with the
Church of Rome, the consolation of beauty so sublime that it
burned away all dogma. Now it was just cold stone, and
beauty an apparition that had deserted me.

We were much better off on the open road, winding from
village to village, picnicking under the drowse of sycamores,
the brown fields like a harvest quilt. Lazily Craig unfolded our
vast Italian road map, a double accordian, finding the exact
spot where we sat finishing our pears and nougat, quickly before the bees gathered. Craig trailed a finger along the Tiber
where it cleaved the north country in two. "What's on the
other side of the river?" he asked.

"Umbria," I replied with some indifference. We were due
to fly out of Rome day after next, and all I wanted now was
to get back home to Puck and to Roger's grave. But I peered
at the map and lighted upon Assisi, which looked to be about
a hundred kilometers away. "You want to drive over there for
the night?" Even I could hear the longing in my voice.

"Is it all churches?" he wondered cautiously.

"Oh no," I replied, a brazen lie, since I hadn't the first
idea what was there. Maybe a cross to mark the spot where
Francis preached to the birds, which was about all I knew of
the life of the saint.

We set off at once, into a swirling mist that became a
driving downpour as we crossed into Umbria. Craig grew
grumpy and curled asleep. The single windshield wiper did no
more than smear the rain. What I'd thought we could do in
two hours stretched to four, and I was verging on a panic

attack, wondering what the fuck I was doing. All I could think was I'd never been there—a totally new place, unspoiled by what Roger had once called "the drag of nostalgia."

We snaked our way up the mountain, the road a torrent. Because of the low-hung clouds we couldn't see two feet ahead as we found our dank hotel. It was ten minutes to five, night already. The desk clerk told us the Basilica of Saint Francis was open till five-fifteen, and only a hundred feet away. "You better go see it," Craig ordered me dryly, eager himself to get to the room and collapse. So I set off into the flood, umbrella-less, leaping puddles till I came to the doors of the lower church. The Basilica is a double decker, the lower church much more gloomy and claustrophobic, but containing the actual tomb of the saint. Shaking off the rain like a dog, I stopped in the first chapel, where under glass was displayed Francis's brown hooded tunic, patched in a dozen places. The vow of poverty so physical you could almost touch it.

Turning to go, I was startled to see a young monk watching me—his own brown robe exactly the same as the saint's, no fashion changes having been deemed necessary in the intervening seven hundred years. I brushed past him, eyes downcast, not wishing to intrude upon his prayers, then made my way toward the tomb, feeding the two-hundred *lire* slots along the wall to light up the frescoes. The place was empty, and perhaps that explained how hyperaware I was of the monk padding along in my wake.

But I hardly gave it a second thought, figuring him to be a species of guard making sure I didn't purloin a candlestick. I descended into the crypt below the altar, where the sarcophagus lies enclosed by a kind of prison grille to protect it. It was so cold down there that my teeth began to rattle. I headed back to the stairs, suddenly wanting out—but was stopped in my tracks by the sentry posture of the young monk, smiling curiously at me from the bottom step. I nodded politely but had no Italian to small-talk past him. He lifted an eyebrow and pursed a funny grin, swaying a bit inside his robe. If this was a spiritual posture, then I was the Bishop of Rome. He was *cruising* me.

I drew myself up with unconcealed contempt, offended somehow for Francis's sake. The monk only leered more openly. It wasn't a sacrilege against anything I believed. In fact I should have been crowing at such a pure example of the rot at the heart of piety. What did he want us to do, dart behind the sarcophagus so he could give me a blow job? He was waiting for me to make the next move. He lounged against the banister, coquettish and yet oddly passive, a virgin tramp. Giving him nothing back, I left by the opposite staircase, as huffy as a Puritan divine.

"Well, was he *cute?*" asked Craig when I got back to the hotel.

"I don't know, I guess if you like them hooded. He was *creepy.*"

"Some people," he drawled, "would give their left nut to be done by a monk in a crypt."

Thus did we laugh it off and gorge ourselves on Parma ham and pasta. But as I lay there waiting to sleep, long after midnight, restless from the drumming of the rain on the red tile roofs, I berated myself for having been so icily aloof. I could have ignored his clumsy advance and still been kind, acknowledging we were brothers somehow. I even knew what it was that had made me cruel: how much his awkward pose and tentative pass had called back my own ineffectual moves at twenty-five, eyeing men from a hopeless distance. Always terrified that one of them would respond in kind, giving me back what I wanted and dared not have. I had acted out instead the affronted pride of a straight man.

The morning broke in a blaze of gold. Craig, a very slow riser, banished me to an hour's shopping while he took a bath. He wanted Assisi souvenirs even if he hadn't caught a glimpse of the place himself. As soon as I stepped outside it grabbed me: the whole town built of the rosy-ochre local stone, a revelation after the night and the rain. I bought a guidebook and raced to the main square, speed-reading Francis's story as I went. I found the spot where he renounced his father, stripping himself naked in the plaza and giving up the garments of a young nobleman. I gazed up the pinnacle slopes of Mount Subasio to where he'd lived in the caves with his followers. The day was unearthly bright, the window boxes all through the town still glutted with flowers, no frost yet. The views out over the Umbrian plain were unlike anything in my lifelong travelogue—something new at last. A pagan beauty restored, like a gift of second sight.

By the time I joined Craig for rolls and cappuccino, I was fairly babbling over the glories of Assisi. I'd stumbled onto the Church of Saint Clare, Sister Moon to Francis's Brother Sun. Her personal best involved an army of Huns or Visigoths bearing across the flood plain, a thunder of horses and brandished swords. Clare grabbed a monstrance containing the Host and strode down the mountain, holding the Blessed Sacrament before her like another kind of sword. She marched across the plain toward the advancing army, and the light caught the Host, blinding the soldiers and bringing them to a dead halt. Clare did not retreat. The invading army turned and ran.

Right on, Clare! As I told the tale to Craig, there was no question in my mind that Clare and Francis were queer. She bestrode the wilderness like Diana the Huntress, her pagan forebear, while her eremite brother communed with the birds and flowers, Pan in a patched cloak. "Okay, okay," Craig replied, but where were his postcards and tee-shirt? If we didn't leave right now, he fretted, we might not make Rome till after dark, where we had no reservation.

Just look at *something,* I pleaded with him, coaxing him at last to a quick duck into the basilica. He looked impassively at the frescoes, as clear to me now as news footage, so well had

I drunk up the stories since my visit in the dark. I was giving a mini-lecture about one of the Giottos when Craig bumped my shoulder. "Is that him?"

Perplexed, I followed his most unsubtle stare. And there was the monk from the night before, startled to see me again and uncertain whether to smile or nod. For all I knew he'd been to confession since the incident, and was even now praying his penance. "He *is* cute," Craig observed, making no effort to keep his voice low, the dish reverberating across the vaulting stones. The monk glanced at Craig and then me, his face gone blank but hiding nothing. Either he felt betrayed that I'd told his sin, or he ached to see the two of us together—so casually fraternal, without any secrets. I didn't know what to do, and then he had turned away, an old man's stoop in his shoulders as he padded off. I felt that I was the one who'd sinned.

So what is a pilgimage anyway? I suppose it has to do with the baggage you carry and the baggage you manage to shed. Almost by definition, the reality is the opposite of your expectations—or why go at all? Faith is the driving force that makes Crusades. In Henry Adams's brilliant formulation, *The Virgin and the Dynamo,* he makes clear that no modern engineering could have built Chartres. The sublime of it could only be achieved by the fervor of belief, stone patiently fitted to stone for two hundred years till the steeples were finally topped.

I went to Assisi without belief and left it much the same, without stigmata, untransformed. But buoyed all the same by its memories, by that medieval fortitude that filled the hearts of its saints. And by the sight of that one frightened monk grappling with his vows, enslaved by a chain of command that went all the way to the Vatican. He is the reason I've come to think Jerry Silver had it exactly right, with his hundred-and-ten percent. A whole army of self-loathing men, estranged from women, estranged from the life of the body—did they really mean to go into a system so bankrupt, so inhuman, that it dares to declare as policy that getting AIDS is preferable to wearing a condom?

In memory it's all mixed up, the saint among the Giotto frescoes and the disconnected queer. If I wasn't changed, then maybe the young monk was. Beauty was what I had grown bereft of, and Assisi managed to give it back. Perhaps that's more of a transformation than I realize, if not exactly the transfiguring kind. In any case my invective against the Church hasn't moderated perceptibly, but I try to focus the laser of my rage where the power is, on the Roman-collared politicians.

Yet I understand that on some level all religion is local— just like politics: wards and precincts. Two days after Christmas in '86, my friend Star and I drove north from Albuquerque, three hours into the desert. We came to a pueblo village miles from anywhere, a few dozen adobe and tarpaper houses grouped about a dusty plaza. We'd come to see the dancing, and as it happened we were the only two non-natives there that day. There were closer villages, after all, with well-worn tourist tracks. The women who hurried out to greet us couldn't have been more delighted, beckoning us impatiently to follow, as if we were missing the best part.

It was the men who danced in the plaza, a long sinewy line of them drumming their feet on the ground, clowns darting among them. This was the dance that D. H. Lawrence said transformed the earth itself into a drumskin, noting that these dancers had been beating the ground for thousands of years before the conquerors came with their crosses. Lawrence had no doubt, witnessing the ceremony, that they would be dancing a thousand years hence, long after the last white men had vanished. In the bone chill of the setting sun, a zero wind blowing in from Chaco Mesa, I thought how close we were to Los Alamos, where whole millennia had collapsed in the quonset labs of the Manhattan Project. A bare few hours north of Alamogordo itself, where a different sort of zero had been reached. And still the Indians danced.

As dusk fell, the Christmas lights went on in several of the houses—back-lit Santas in the windows, cartoon dioramas of Mary and Joseph winding their way to Bethlehem, the Virgin on a donkey. Which was their religion, I wondered—the spirit power of the Old Ones, or the Christian mishmash? They couldn't have it both ways—or could they? All that seemed to remain of the missionary padres were the strings of colored lights. No Christian priest marred this solstice ceremony, raining them with holy water. The real religion was deeper down, so local it vibrated only here on this quaking ground. And yet, so universal is the particular, that its echoing force on the plaza at Santo Domingo was like Thoreau's wildflower. You plucked it, and the whole universe came with it.

I thought I had severed my own local affiliations long ago, by ceasing to believe. It was sentiment more than anything that brought me back every Christmas to an Episcopal church on Hollywood Boulevard, whose gray stone and polished oak reminded me of New England. Its regular parishioners seemed to number around thirty, widows in hats and white gloves, barely sufficient to pay the gas and electric, I would've thought. On Christmas Eve it swelled a bit, but you'd hardly call it a crowd. I would put my ten bucks in the plate for the privilege of singing carols, wanting no ministrations. So perverse was I—so conflicted, I suppose—that when my mother would call on Christmas Day, plaintively asking if I'd managed to make it to church the night before, "for the singing," I curtly answered "No." Not wanting her to get the wrong idea that I'd had a sudden change of heart.

Then about seven years ago they hired a new rector at Saint Thomas the Apostle. I never heard a word about it till much later, and first saw Father Carroll himself the following Christmas Eve. Apparently, right from the first, he'd been

speaking positive thoughts from the pulpit about gay and lesbian people, and thus had roused the ire of a "family" man. A
fourth-rate actor with jowls that flapped when he got on his
high horse, who was damned if he'd let his children be fouled
by such rank blasphemy. A storm of protest rocked the parish
council, reaching all the way to the Bishop, egged on by this
lowlife porker. Finally it was suggested that he and his family
might be happier in another parish.

All I could see, on my Christmas visits, was that Saint
Thomas was more and more crowded, especially with queers.
Father Carroll was very high-church, startling to me who'd
never choked on incense before, not in the low church of my
youth. For the first time ever I experienced a service sung in
plainchant. I heard Father Carroll had opened the door to Dignity, the gay and lesbian Catholic group who'd been banished
from all church property by Cardinal Mahony. Saint Thomas
dedicated an AIDS chapel, with a book of names on the altar.
AIDS memorial services became standard fare, as well as a
myriad of support groups for those in the grip of HIV.

I was proud of all that, and sent checks to support Father
Carroll's work. His assistant rector died of AIDS a couple of
years later, and then his own son. He's been through the fire.
And over the course of time we've developed a certain unde-
manding acquaintance, Father Carroll and I. He looks politely
puzzled when I tell him I'm an atheist who's still a card-
carrying Episcopalian. My mother, were she still alive, would
welcome all this as a sort of prodigal return to the faith of my
fathers—but then I'd probably keep the details from her still.
When I had a letter some years ago from the Presiding Bishop
in New York, head of the church in America, promising
greater outreach in the fight against AIDS discrimination, my
mother was beside herself for months. It might have been a
letter from Jesus himself.

But for all their liberal eloquence and their wide open
doors, *have* they done enough? I remember replying to Bishop

Browning's letter with a query of my own. What was it like, I asked, trying not to be flippant, to mix it up with the other faiths at the National Council of Churches? Did they all play golf together? At the prayer breakfasts, did he bow his head in unison with preachers who wanted my people dead? It seemed to me that hatred of queers was at the very top of the list for most religions. So what did it mean to serve witness to the power of love if the hate was never challenged? The National Council ought to be a brawl, not just more tepid lip-service to ecumenism and One God. Christ, whatever he was, was not about breakfasts.

I had a surprise visit not long ago from another Episcopal Bishop, this one from the Midwest. He was passing through L.A. and wondered if we might have a cup of tea. I readily agreed, having just begun these reflections. He was strikingly handsome, with a full head of white hair—and dressed in civvies, to Winston's disappointment, who'd rather hoped for a miter and crozier. But the Bishop was very down-to-earth, no standing on ceremony. He openly admitted to being gay, out to himself for almost twenty years, and out to his wife and children too, the marriage having survived the revelation. Now he was nearly seventy years old, about to retire, and beginning to ready himself for the pilgrimage (his word) of his life's next phase. No one in his ministry knew his secret—a conscious choice, apparently, so as not to bring controversy to the institution.

But he knew he hadn't done enough. Just as it wasn't enough that a third woman has recently been elevated to the House of Bishops. Better, the Bishop allowed, but two hundred years late. Meanwhile I have no idea if he's ever acted on his queer impulses—lying down with a man—but it was certainly clear to Winston and me that he wanted out of the closet, to march unfettered with his gay brothers and sisters. I suggested he work to put gay and lesbian issues into the seminary curricula, and to keep the pressure on to bring queers

into the ministry. Winston, more daring than I, advised the
Bishop to stand at the next House meeting and come out publicly. That ought to shake their miters.

He gave us the most benign and thoughtful gaze. (So in-
finitely discreet had been his life.) He nodded and said he'd
consider it—beginning to see, I think, how many miles you
could travel in a single step. At the end he asked if I would
consider giving some writerly input to the church's task of
composing a commitment ceremony for gay and lesbian cou-
ples. Auden, he said, had helped with the recent moderniza-
tion of the King James prayer book—a bad job, I'd always
thought, flattening out all the gorgeous Shakespearean locu-
tions of the original. Did that mean I was a *conservative* Episcopalian atheist, kin to those retrograde Catholics who swear it's
never been the same since they took the Latin away?

"We don't *need* their commitment service," counters Malcolm Boyd, who took off his own mask a quarter century ago.
A priest who donned the collar so he could join the fight for
justice in Selma and Little Rock, who'd been challenging the
church's homophobia since I was a kid. "Why? So we can
have marriages as screwed-up as theirs? We deserve better than
scraps."

Iconoclast and gadfly—that's Malcolm. He can't abide the
noblesse oblige of the Lincoln Town Car Protestants. In his own
meditations and books of prayer, he wrestles God as Jacob
wrestled the angel, till the breaking of the day. It would be
inconceivable to him to wear the collar and *not* take a stand
on the gathering rubble of the American empire, where justice
is mostly a business expense, cheap at the price. To be a priest
and stay in the closet, according to Malcolm, is to forfeit the
moral center and live a coward's half-life besides, accepting the
scraps of internal exile. In his own life he had experienced an
overflow of love, a long and healing relationship with Mark
Thompson, his comrade of the heart. That bonding was its
own blessing, requiring no official stamp. Indeed, Malcolm and

Mark are the perfect marriage of Christian and pagan, priest and shaman, a balance of souls that neutralized all dogma.

I leave it to my fellow queer Episcopalians to fight for a special service, if it brings them closer to what Tillich calls "the ground of being." Wear white from Priscilla of Boston with an eight-foot train and illusion veil, if it feels right. As it happens, Winston and I do not require the blessing of the church—for any number of reasons, but mostly because we're already married. Last April. Ma officiated.

Ma is something else. A guru from Brooklyn who has never lost her stevedore's swagger or street tough's lip. She runs an ashram in Florida, with eighty or a hundred in permanent residence, and a constant flow of pilgrims. She would call herself a Hindu—I think—but her teachings cast a very wide net. Tattoos peek through her saris, and she has enough piercings and bangles to set off the alarms at LAX. A caste mark on her forehead, Revlon bright.

But it was some months before I saw any of that. Stevie was in his last summer when the first calls came, messages left by one of Ma's lieutenants asking me to come by and meet her: "You mean a lot to her." I balked. I'd struggled with the various denial systems purveyed by a raft of New Age gurus, the ones who filled whole auditoriums in Hollywood, promising that if we loved ourselves enough we wouldn't die. Tapes available at the door, $29.95, no checks please. Courses in miracles, follow the white light, anger will kill you faster than AIDS. Et cetera.

The worst. Designed to make people feel that if they *did* get sicker, they weren't loving their lesions enough, or keeping up with their positive imaging. In a word, the dying were losers. I had watched too many acquaintances, gulled into fairyland by Louise and Marianne, turn bitterly away from them when the disease began to win. The New Age ladies drew the line at visiting the dying. Play those tapes, boys, louder and louder. My neighbor Billy, who'd gloried in his role as Ed McMahon to the Wednesday evening "Hayrides," went into a black depression when the lesions swarmed over his face. The New Age stopped returning his calls. He hanged himself from the clothes bar in his closet, undiscovered for three days, till a pair of lesbian friends from back East arrived for the weekend and broke down the door.

I was not in the market for gurus, thanks. By the time Ma's people called again, about three months later, Stevie had been dead a week and I was stiff as a corpse myself, staring at the ceiling. I was given to understand that Ma made regular visits to Los Angeles four times a year, taking over the house of one of her disciples and welcoming people in, especially those with HIV.

"But what does she *do,* exactly?" I asked in some confusion.

I could hear the shrug through the phone, as if there were things that didn't translate into words. "She teaches," came the reply at last. "Your book is very important to her."

A bungalow south of Melrose—tidy little front yards all up and down the street till you got to Ma's place, where the overflow of pilgrims spilled out and sprawled in the grass. The porch was a heap of shoes, because you were meant to walk unshod into the presence of the guru. Inside there were men curled up on the floor on straw mats, clearly in the very last stages. Others slumped in wheelchairs. But the prevailing mood was holiday bustle, as several long-haired types in harlequin deshabille bore platters to the groaning board of the vegetarian feast, for three days of feeding round the clock. No evidence, as at Lourdes, that anyone had flung his crutches aside, healed by faith. Nothing, in fact, that smacked of religion.

They led me in to see her, sitting in lotus on a wicker chair, more veils than Salome, though none to cover her beaming face. As soon as she saw me she shrieked in Brooklynese to the twenty or thirty disciples who jammed the little bedroom: "All right, now nobody mention God! He doesn't want to hear that crap!"

Then I was enfolded in her embrace as she brayed with excitement, calling in more and more people till we were like sardines in there. "This is the man who wrote my Bible," she announced with a gush of pride, then made me sit on a chair face to face with her while the others sat cross-legged on the floor. She told me how she visited the county homes in Florida, where the most wretched of those with AIDS were taken to die. Many of these had been abandoned by their families, denied the comforts of "traditional" religions. And Ma crawled into bed with them and kissed their lesions. Her raucous guttersnipe's laugh preceded her down the puke-green corridors as the dying perked up to greet her. She came to them completely unafraid of death, honored in fact to be in its presence, and gave them all a bluesy sort of comfort. Without the God crap.

Ma worries that I paint too bleak a picture of the county homes—which aren't so bad, Bina assures me, run by dedicated and compassionate staff. My own theory is that if it's not so bleak, it's because Ma's presence has changed these places, given them life. Apparently she often reads aloud from *Borrowed Time,* especially the parts that tell about loving till the very end, the minor victories: a walk to the corner, a good foot rub. I don't know if Ma understands that the book and I are not the same, or to put it another way, that I'm not remotely as wise as the book. Not that I'm being humble—a feeling my friends would never accuse me of—but rather that I have a sense of the book's own journey, the dark places where it can go and I can't.

The bedside of a frightened man of color, for instance— hardly a bag of bones as he arched against the pain. He loved to hear Ma read about me and Roger, almost a folk tale to him. "I wish I had one of my own," he sighed, meaning the book. "But you can't read, can you?" retorted Ma. Illiterate all his life, and almost blind besides, he shrugged, like Bina over the phone when I asked her what Ma did. She handed him her copy.

It was his prize possession, apparently, from that day on. His *only* possession, Ma would be quick to tell you, there in the death camp of Palm Beach County. And just before he went a few weeks later, he summoned a nurse so he could dictate his will. She must've thought it was the dementia creeping up, but humored him by getting paper and pen. "I leave my book of *Borrowed Time*," he whispered, "to anyone who can read." Signed with an X and duly witnessed.

Who is the priest here? Where is God exactly? Don't look at me. These deathbed wills are like those Christmas trees at Starcross—they'd throw you out of the Iowa Writers' Workshop on your ear if you tried to pass it off as fiction. I admit to a certain amount of religion by association, but for healing purposes the touch and the teaching are all Ma. I am just a useful text. If people get restless during a group audience, chatting among themselves as they shift their aching knees, she is liable to bellow for silence. "I'm the holy mother around here," she squalls. "And there's only room for one, so shut up and listen." The Auntie Mame of gurus.

Winston took to coming with me when I made my seasonal visits, figuring this was the nearest he would see me in a spiritual mode (if you don't count ripping up the Pontiff's picture, which I do out of solidarity with Sinead). Ma embraced us both. We didn't stay for *darshan,* her hour of public teaching in a rented tent in the back yard. I made my salutations and withdrew, more out of respect for her than for a faith I didn't share: But when, one Sunday afternoon in spring, Ma happened to mention in passing that she'd married a lesbian couple the night before—well, it seemed the most natural thing to ask her to bless us too.

Ma is emphatically not the sort of person you have to ask

twice. Scarcely pausing for breath, she drew our hands together and held our eyes with hers—"Look at the dot"—as
she spun the ritual out of her heart. Seemingly impromptu, but
then blessing is what Ma does. Word spread quickly among the
assembled disciples and pilgrims, and they all hugged us joy-
fully and led us out to the driveway feast. Ma introduced Win-
nie and me and the lesbians at *darshan*—we made an exception
and stayed that night—and Arlo sang us a wedding song.

No time to register at Geary's or send out Tiffany invites.
All our friends would hear about it after the fact, some of
them crushed not to be included. But they quickly came to
understand that it was the right sort of wedding for us. In the
pictures taken that day, we are shawled in perfumed scarves
and grinning, as if we'd been showered by a couple of wayward angels. No priest in evidence. Perhaps the faintest sound
of drumming.

Seven months later it's Saturnalia, the pagan turn of the
year, under an ink-blue sky awash in stars, cold enough for a
topcoat even here in L.A. For what is shaping up to be my
last Christmas—oh well, my *second*-to-last then, denial being
intrinsic to the ho-ho of the season—I'm pulling out all the
stops, but not for Baby Jesus's sake. The tree from Starcross is
up in the living room, decked and gleaming, as well as a
wreath on the front door, the latter sent gratis by Toby and
the sisters because I'm their friend. Tomorrow night we'll be
going to St. Thomas for the singing. I will take a small vacation from my hammering at the Vatican, like a ceasefire over
enemy lines, a prayer for peace in a babel of tongues. The
fighting will start up again next week.

At Gucci in Rome, the fur account of the Vatican is said
to be the largest of all—those ermine shrugs and sable-lined
dressing gowns, chinchilla throws on the daybeds, millions and
millions of lire to keep the tyrants cozy, the emperors of God.
Meanwhile Gambone, my ex-Jesuit, writes to tell me he's off

to a cabin in the northern Minnesota wilds, to figure out the next step. Father Tom is readying for a season in Rome, to grapple with the hateful dogmas—or to find love, he isn't sure which himself. At the spring convocation, the Bishop just might stand up and declare himself. Or the volunteer firemen in Santa Rosa may show up for the next emergency, gloved and masked to be sure, but determined to save a baby's life.

There is no God, I'm sure of that. But the more they've sought me out, the more convinced I am that there *are* holy men and women. So I send blessings, such as they are, to all my priests who constitute the Resistance. Down with the fur and the edicts. And if they like, they're welcome to include me in their prayers. Can't hurt. None of us will free the world of intolerance alone. We need the people of God, especially if He isn't there.

3275

THERE ARE TWO perfect graves. Well, actually three, but I haven't the wherewithal or the strength these days to travel as far as Samoa. Stevenson himself was sicker than I when he made his voyage there, a last-ditch flight to paradise. Or did he see it as his own *Treasure Island* at last, a chance to consult with parrots and pegleg castaways? Free from Edwardian clutter and the satanic mills of England, perhaps he expected to stumble on a pirate's map. Which in turn would lead him to a sheltered cove, the strongbox hidden in a sea cave whose entrance lay underwater except at the ebb of lowest tide. A boy's adventure for a dying man, hammocked in coconut shade as his own strength ebbed.

His grave is on a promontory overlooking a thousand miles of ocean, so vast you can see the curve of the planet, but maybe that's another boy's illusion. Cut into the slab of stone—granite? quarried where?—is what amounts to the granddaddy of fin-de-siècle epitaphs:

THIS BE THE VERSE YOU GRAVE FOR ME:
HERE HE LIES WHERE HE LONGED TO BE;
HOME IS THE SAILOR, HOME FROM SEA,
    AND THE HUNTER HOME FROM THE HILL.

Exquisite, that use of "grave" for "engrave," as if the action of the stonecutter and the place itself are one. A lookout, surely, worth a journey halfway round the world. I can see myself there, one foot planted on Stevenson's brow, the trade wind billowing my sailor's blouse as I lift my brassbound spyglass and comb the lordly Pacific. My very own *National Geographic* special.

But not to be realized in the flesh, not in my time anyway. I leave it to stauncher travelers to make the trek to Stevenson's summit, there perhaps to deconstruct the romantic gush of fantasies like mine. Happily no one can desecrate or diminish my other two totems, because I've actually been to them. To the snowbound chapel where Lawrence is buried, in the Sangre de Cristo foothills, on a perch that looks across the high desert beyond the Rio Grande all the way to Arizona. And to the Protestant Cemetery in Rome, where Keats is buried with a half-strung lyre on his tombstone and that final statement written in fire. Surrounded by a meadow of shaggy grass, electric-green, an echo of England in April, the spring that never arrived for the choking poet.

It's only half-true to say that I became a seeker of graves because of AIDS. I grew up in a town pocked with graveyards, old church burial-grounds whose tilted slates have long since lost their graven names. Even then as a melancholy boy I'd sit on a stone, chin in hand, and contemplate the cosmos. Or these country graveyards fenced in iron staves and overhung with willows, the family plot no bigger than a farmhouse bedroom. If they were meant to be a *memento mori*, it was all unconscious to me. Though I daresay I looked like a spook out of Edward Gorey, I don't remember ruminating on death exactly. Rather they constituted a sort of safety zone, where I could indulge my secret longing to be a poet, the chokeless kind.

The first grave I ever tracked down for writerly reasons was Edmund Wilson's. Nothing personal. I'd read an account of the woodland spot where he lay buried with all his honors. A discreet white marble slab two feet high, rounded at the top like the curve of grief itself, and bearing beneath the writer's name three Hebrew letters, which, roughly translated, exhorted the scholar's soul to *Go on from strength to strength*. I carried all of this on a tattered newspaper clipping in my wallet, waiting for the next trip Roger and I made to Provincetown.

The village of Wellfleet is hardly even a detour, the Cape is so narrow beyond the elbow. We found the hillside graveyard without any map or questions asked. Wilson is off by himself under the trees, and it happened that a single daffodil bloomed yellow in front of the stone. It is a detail which at the time cheered me immensely, the opposite of a wilting bouquet, the widow's work of planting a bulb like spitting in Death's face. Mixed up in my head by then—stuffed as it was by overeducation—were fragments of Gray's "Elegy in a Country Churchyard" and Lowell's "Quaker Graveyard in Nantucket." But all of it was still in the realm of the picturesque, no muffled echo of a bell that tolled for me. If anything, this high literary take on darkness managed to push the thing itself away, an amulet of prettied-up quotes safely recorded in Bartlett's.

One visited such places politely, if not piously—like Harold and Maude attending the funerals of strangers, transported by the organ prelude and checking out everyone's hat. Trying on other people's survivors like so many veils, and underneath it all learning how to cry. The first public event I went to after moving to L.A. was Howard Hawks's funeral. I didn't know anyone there, couldn't even have said what movies the man had directed. But I sat next to Angie Dickinson, feeling quite swank, and listened with rapt attention as John Wayne gave the eulogy. I felt faintly ashamed afterward, dissatisfied and incomplete, the way I used to feel in the closet. Thereafter I avoided the obsequies of stars.

Then in the fall of '83 Roger and I were in Rome, having wound our way through Tuscany, waiting overnight to catch a plane back to L.A. We only had a single free afternoon, and decided to track down the Keats-Shelley Memorial House, overlooking the Spanish Steps. A most fusty and eccentric place, chockablock with memorabilia in the Victorian manner, cut-paper silhouettes and locks of everyone's hair. The whole presided over by a sunken-cheeked vicar who didn't appear to want visitors at all.

It took us a while to get our bearings, no help from the vicar. But soon we were reading Joseph Severn's diary under glass, a rending account of the poet's last days. We realized that the tiny room in the front corner was where Keats had actually died, with a window onto the Steps and the Bernini fountain in the piazza. Bernini's conceit was a simple stone boat with gouts of water pouring from its sides, a leaky vessel the sound of whose plashing reached us in the death-room. By all accounts the poet in his final hours was calm and resigned, though agitated at the end by a letter from Fanny Brawne which he couldn't bring himself to open, much less read. He asked that Severn place it in the folds of his winding sheet.

And then that final night, Severn sketching beside the bed to keep himself from going mad with grief. *28 Janry 3 o'clock mng,* he has scrawled in charcoal beneath the sketch of the poet's head lolling on a pillow. *Drawn to keep me awake, a deadly sweat was on him all this night.* And framed above the glass cabinet of Severn's memory, an artist's ink drawing of the grave they bore him to. You couldn't get through college English, in my time anyway, without some passing reference to the name that was *writ in water*. But somehow the full text had escaped me until now, and it brought me up extremely short.

THIS GRAVE

CONTAINS ALL THAT WAS MORTAL

OF A

YOUNG ENGLISH POET,

WHO,

ON HIS DEATH BED,

IN THE BITTERNESS OF HIS HEART,

AT THE MALICIOUS POWER OF HIS ENEMIES,

DESIRED

THESE WORDS TO BE ENGRAVEN ON HIS TOMB STONE:

"HERE LIES ONE
WHOSE NAME WAS WRIT IN WATER."

FEB 21ST, 1821

I turned to Roger and said with a kind of fevered resolve: "We have to go there. Right now."

But it was already growing dusk in the piazza below, nearly five o'clock and the vicar squirming to be rid of us. The Protestant Cemetery was too far away, its gates padlocked at nightfall. No time in the morning either, since we had to be up at dawn to make the airport. "Next trip," I said to myself, dissatisfied and suddenly full of portent, a shiver of mortality and the roads that don't lead back.

At the time I was feeling not a little *writ in water* myself, a novel of mine having been savaged by a couple of reviewers in the gay press. One had called me up from Philadelphia and asked, "Is everyone in California as shallow as the characters

in your books?" Another in the *New York Native* had opined
that someone had to put a stop to dickless, no-talent writers
like me, who were keeping good work from being
published—wasting the trees, as it were. Since nobody in the
"mainstream" press paid any attention to any of us, these scab-
rous ·remarks constituted the record regarding my work.
Which was, in any case, completely out of print within another year. For a long while my confidence was shot, my next
novel rejected by thirty publishers. I tended the bitterness of
my heart. Worse, I was hip-deep in malarial waters on which
I wrote my own name in the scum—Hollywood, I mean.
Hardly a worthy comparison to the silencing of the finest lyric
voice in English poetry, but there you are. Sometimes all you
have left as an artist is histrionics.

Somewhere in there, in the winter after Italy, I conceived
the reckless scheme of writing a play about Keats's final week.
A nine-days'-wonder of a notion, to take place in that very
apartment above the Spanish Steps. With Severn and a landlady to care for him, and the landlady's ripe peasant daughter
bringing up milk and hearty soups. *My* conceit was that the
poet, delirious in the throes of fever, would come to think the
landlady's daughter was Fanny Brawne herself, to whom he
would declare his undying love through the rattle of his
drowning lungs. I imagined a visit by members of the Milton
Society, lovers of Poesy, fawning at Keats's bedside though
managing all the while to cover their noses and mouths with
handkerchiefs. I was going to have Keats cough desperately to
scare them away. And to vary the setting I'd show the outing
Keats and Severn made to the Protestant Cemetery, before the
poet was too ill to leave his bed. The meadow was pocked
with violets that day. Keats sighed when he saw them, expressing a longing to pull the cover of grass over him, so the violets
would carpet his heart.

But I only got as far as checking the books out of the

library. By the time I'd read twenty pages of Walter Jackson
Bates's huge biography, weighty as a tombstone itself, my eyes
had glazed over. I was never any good at research—not
blessed with that punctilious turn of mind that orders the
world on three-by-five cards. I couldn't even say where the
details come from here as I write them down, what's "true"
and what's romantic license. I haven't a footnote in my head.
Besides, how had I ever expected to get away with writing
proper English speech, let alone broken Italian, not to mention
nineteenth-century voices that didn't sound like community
theater? I blew the whole thing off my desk. Let John Keats
die in peace.

Before another year was out, all my friends were dying
instead. But by some quirk of coincidence, none of them was
buried in a cemetery. Scattered ashes and memorial services
were the fashion, all too often without any reference to AIDS
or even gay. We let loose our balloons and made a final circuit
through the house of the deceased—where the final battle was
already taking place between the "blood" family and the lover,
fighting over the towels and the lamps and the bibelots.

The morning after Roger died, his half-brother came bustling into my room and stirred me from my Dalmane twilight.
"You've got work to do," he said, and when I frowned in
confusion, added, "Where's he going? You've got to pick a
place."

The Protestant Cemetery in Rome, I thought irrelevantly, sitting slumped in the back of the car as we toured the city's
cemeteries. When we got to Forest Lawn, Hollywood Hills
division, the only thing left in my heart besides the grief was
a horror of finding myself in *The Loved One.* For this was
surely the very place envisioned by Waugh—the sweep of
grass like a Palm Springs golf course, no gravestones permitted,
only bronze plaques in the ground. Nothing to mar the founder's vision of a Park of Death, joyous with children playing

and family picnics, all the dead having gone to heaven. Anchored at one end by a white clapboard village church, or at least the Disney equivalent, and on the other by a half-scale replica of the Old North Church in Boston, of course with generous parking. Dotted about the landscape were white marble statues of stupefying vulgarity, Moms and Dads and kids in frozen groups, little tykes on their knees praying.

But at least no Jesus shit that I could detect. And as it turned out, when we entered the Tara reception center, the theme of the Hollywood Hills division was God Bless America—a garden of patriots as its centerpiece, full-scale bronzes of Washington and Jefferson, and a huge outdoor mural of the signing of the Declaration. Hallmark meets *My Weekly Reader.* Our Comfort Counselor, Mr. Wheeler, was not quite Rod Steiger in a powdered wig, though his nails were lugubriously clean. He moved in a cloud of Aramis that stung the eyes within ten feet of him.

Real estate came first, as it always does in California. Roger's parents and I were driven about in Mr. Wheeler's Cadillac, two miles an hour, as he pointed out each section from Heavenly Rest to Resurrection. I directed him up the winding hill to the highest plots, where the lawn verged on undeveloped chaparral. Atheists all, we abandoned the car and trudged uphill in Mr. Wheeler's wake, the hillside shaded by umbrella pines and with a view across the valley to the San Bernardinos if the smog was light. Wheeler carried a big book like a survey map, the whole acreage divided into numbered plots.

They were sold in pairs, side by side. Puffing from the climb, we decided we liked where we were. A deal: Plot 3275, Spaces 1 and 2, on the hill called Revelation. Delicately Wheeler inquired which space I wanted Roger in. I shrugged. What did it matter? Roger's mother touched my arm and said, "He wants to know which side you boys slept on in bed." Oh. As a matter of fact it went either way, depending on who needed to be closest to the alarm clock. Let Roger have the right side then. "Excellent," said Mr. Wheeler, circling it on his chart. Then, offhandedly, "This section used to be reserved just for Mormons, but we've opened it up."

I looked around in dismay, only now picking out the Mormon Temple engraved on several bronzes. "Hey, this isn't going to work, Mr. Wheeler. They don't want *us* up here."

He was shocked. "We're all one family in death," I think he said, and I let it go for the parents' sake. "One thing I should tell you, though," he continued. "At night the deer come down and steal the flowers. We can't stop them." He pointed with dismay to the undeveloped scrub on the hillside above, clearly an affront to the manicured lawns of the dead. "Some people don't like it, having their flowers scattered. Sometimes we have to move their loved ones further down the hill. The deer will only go so far."

Al and Bernice were sporting the same dreamy smile I was. "Don't worry, Mr. Wheeler," I assured him. "We like the deer just fine. What kind of flowers do they prefer?"

He gave a bewildered shrug. His expertise lay elsewhere, in the coffin-and-hearse department. By week's end we had buried Roger there, and I still didn't understand that I'd bought the spot where I'd be spending most of the next year and a half.

There was no place else to go, really. Friends would call with an invitation to lunch, or an extra ticket to the Philharmonic, in one ear and out the other. Not that I wasn't grateful to pass the time, but I knew where I needed to be. Usually from three to five in the afternoon, till closing time. Mostly I sat on my own grave—my permanent side of the bed now—and mostly didn't cry. Cried most of the day and night at home already, so this was my break. Seven days a week. On Saturdays I'd bring up café au lait and croissants at noon and read the paper, just as we always used to do. I'd talk out loud to Roger, reciting him poems. Or I'd lie down and fold my hands across my chest, looking up through the trees and trying to adjust to my last address.

From my perch on the hill I could see the day's funerals, straggling out of the churches. A line of slow cars to the gravesite, the mourners standing in a half circle as the coffin was laid on the lowering hoist, the mounded dirt on either side covered with sheets of Astroturf. They don't do the filling in till after everyone's gone. And I don't know if this constitutes a statistical sample, but almost nobody seemed to wear black anymore. Pastels, a lot of lilac and lavender.

I began to wonder which of the dead had died of AIDS. So I undertook a methodical survey of the whole acreage, moving row by row for the better part of a week, checking out every inscription. At the time there were eighty thousand in residence, with room for another fifty thousand. Here and there I'd find them, young men dead at thirty or thirty-five, with a stray quotation from *Hamlet* or *Pooh*. A silent scattered tribe, the first wave of the plague.

Are you reeling from the mawkishness? Because it gets worse. I had almost made a full circuit by now, having come round again to the western ridge where Roger lay, but still two hundred yards to go. And I realized I had stumbled onto the babies' section. Annabelle, two days old; William Jr., May 25–June 16, 1985. Acres of this, the bronze plaques carved with teddy bears and a lot of Christian singsong. Bronze is not an easy medium to write in, but curiously the clichés seem to help. You learn that it's none of your business what other people choose to memorialize, the inadequate words that mark the scar in their heart.

It takes about six weeks to order the bronze and set it in place. They send you a rubbing of the first casting (a hundred bucks extra), on which I made a myriad of fussy changes. It was finished mid-February and laid in place. I came that day nearly faint with trepidation, fearing somehow the finality, the want of exactly the right word. Or perhaps I'd tried to cram too much in. And still I couldn't say whom it was meant to address, what sort of declaration to the future—as if anyone would even notice it except for an obsessive like me. But here it was, the final word on the final hill. I dropped to my knees and read it through over and over, making sure nothing was off.

ROGER DAVID HORWITZ

1941–1986

MY LITTLE FRIEND

WE SAIL TOGETHER

IF WE SAIL AT ALL

BELOVED SON AND BROTHER

THE WISEST AND JUSTEST AND BEST

The last phrase being Plato's final words on Socrates—in his prison cell, the poison having done its work, history's most compelling argument against capital punishment. But here I'm getting it out of sequence. First came the Christmas crisis, when Forest Lawn relaxes its rule against gaudy tributes and NO ARTIFICIAL FLOWERS. Suddenly the gravesites are decked with Christmas trees and tinsel and wreaths and even battery lights. I'd just begun to get used to the quiet of the place, even looked fondly now on the Old North Church, and here I was confronted by a Macy's load of gewgaws.

I wanted to hide somewhere till Christmas was removed. As it happened, Star and Craig flew out from New York to spend the holiday with me, to get me through it. Star convinced me to take a few days with her over New Year's in New Mexico, where I had never been. "As long as we can visit Lawrence's grave," I replied, setting myself a pilgrimage. The second day we headed north of Taos, blinding sun on the snow, to Kiowa Ranch. Off the road on a rutted track, heading uphill and deep into the trees. To the modest cluster of

ranch buildings, the whole of it deeded to David and Frieda
Lawrence by Mabel Dodge, in exchange for the autograph
manuscript of *Sons and Lovers*.

You must climb a steep hill to reach the chapel, but it
wasn't the altitude pounding my heart. My first glimpse of it
stung my eyes. Simple, more like a stuccoed shed than a
church, because crafted by hand. The rose window above the
door is the hub of a tractor's tire, the one above the altar inside
is a wagon wheel. The altar itself is painted silver, with just
the letters DHL incised on the front. A few painted leaves and
sunflowers by Dorothy Brett, the painter who was their boon
companion, who had to put down her ear trumpet to pick up
her brushes.

But it's so silent up there anyway, just the breeze through
the piñon trees and my blubbering relief. I felt as if I were
standing on the Everest of death. In the warped guestbook
several pilgrims had scribbled notes beside their names: *fellow
pagan; a worshiper of the God of free love.* Then you step out the
door into the delirious vastness of the desert below, all ochre
and streaks of purple, and yes the curve of the earth besides. I
had managed to come to a new place where Roger and I had
never been, without expiring of loneliness. And I had the peculiar feeling that Lawrence had given this view to me, sight-
less himself in the urn of ashes sealed in the altar.

> . . . years, even in the exquisite beauty of Sicily, right
> among the old Greek paganism that still lives there,
> had not shattered the essential Christianity on which
> my character was established. Australia was a sort of
> dream or trance, like being under a spell, the self re-
> maining unchanged . . . Tahiti, in a mere glimpse, re-
> pelled me: and so did California, after a stay of a mere
> few weeks. There seemed a strange brutality in the
> spirit of the western coast, and I felt: O, let me get
> away.

But the moment I saw the brilliant, proud morning shine high up over the deserts of Santa Fe, something stood still in my soul, and I started to attend.[1]

He was the same age as Roger when he died, forty-four, and no more chose this site for himself than Roger had his at Forest Lawn. Yet one couldn't help but anthropomorphize the moment, as if Lawrence were crouched in the chapel's doorway, pointing into the distance—like the dead in *Our Town,* gossiping among themselves as they study the daily rounds of the villagers below. Somehow I was drinking in this vista with DHL at my side, or through him or for him. A strange connectedness at certain graves, as if however briefly one became the ghost of the dead.

We went back to the chapel the next day, by which time I managed the visit without tears. But there was something else going on now, a sudden compulsion to get back to Forest Lawn and *our* place—as if this whole visit were a kind of betrayal, sleeping in somebody else's bed before the funeral meats were cold. Abruptly Star and I left, and I stopped at the first payphone to change my reservation, bringing me back to L.A. that night, which was New Year's Eve.

I raced over to Forest Lawn next morning, full-crazy by now, terrified that Roger's grave might have vanished, or else that it had lost the magic closeness it engendered—the nearest I could get to him now except in dreams. Though still laden with Christmas, the cemetery was practically deserted, everyone staying home today to watch football. I dropped to my knees at 3275, announcing that I was home again. Whimpering rather than crying, I buried a Zuni ring I'd picked up on the plaza in Santa Fe, buried it over his heart.

---

1. *D. H. Lawrence and New Mexico,* Keith Sagar, ed. (Salt Lake City, 1982), page 96.

And then I began to keen, rocking back and forth on my haunches. I realized I was trying to match the sound of Roger's moaning when I arrived in his room at UCLA the day he died. A sound I barely understood at the time, a lament of terrible urgent sorrow, calling out but without any words. The cryptococcus had swelled his brain in the night and stolen his center of speech. "Why is he doing that?" I asked the nurse, but she couldn't say. I asked for a shot to calm his agitation, then realized he could answer me by blinking his eyes when I asked him questions. I called his sister and held the phone to his ear as she talked, and he blinked and blinked.

Now ten weeks later, a stillborn year before me, I finally understand that the bleating sound on that last day was Roger calling my name. Through the pounding in his head, the blindness and the paralysis, all his bodily functions out of control, he had somehow heard me come in. Had waited. And once I understood that, I went mad. My moaning rose to a siren pitch, and I clawed at the grass that covered him. Possessed with a fury to dig the six feet down and tear open the lid and clasp him to me, whatever was left. I don't even know what stopped me—exhaustion, I guess, the utter meaninglessness of anything anymore.

Grief *is* madness—ask anyone who's been there. They will tell you it abates with time, but that's a lie. What drowns you in the first year is a force of solitude and helplessness exactly equal in intensity to the love you had for the one who's gone. Equally passionate, equally intimate. The spaces between the stabs of pain grow longer after a while, but they're empty spaces. The clichés of condolence get you back to the office, back to your taxes and the dinner table—and for everyone else's sake, you collaborate. The road of least resistance is paved with the gravel of well-meaning friends, rather like the gravel that cremation leaves.

Most of my friends would have said I was doing quite well

as we passed the first anniversary. I finished the draft of *Borrowed Time* and set off with Craig for Italy, spending the first night in Rome, just off the Piazza Navona where Roger and I had spent the *last* night of our trip in '83. I had no plans to visit Keats's grave, having given over the sum of my graveyard vigil to 3275. But the jet lag woke me wired at dawn, and Craig was a slower riser even than I. Our train to Florence wasn't leaving till eleven.

I scribbled a note and left on foot, my map of the city blown to shreds by the wind off the Tiber. No taxis in sight, but maybe I just needed to get there on my own. I had no idea what the hours were, and got sidetracked in my confusion by a military cemetery across the way, immaculate and precise as a full-dress drill. A wizened gardener put me right with a lot of gesticulating, and at last I found the crooked side street and the door in the weed-chinked wall.

Open, even so early, and utterly deserted. It seemed at first a typical urban burial-ground, no vacancy and no breathing space, crammed with the marble monuments of another age. But there was a sign nailed to a tree that said KEATS AND SEVERN, with an arrow pointing past the caretaker's office. Beyond that point the tenement crowdedness opened out onto a pristine lawn, only a handful of graves, someone having made a shrewd Protestant decision to stop any further burial here, for Keats's sake perhaps. An acre of green bordered on one side by the Cestius pyramid—erected 16 B.C. The Christian in the shadow of the pagan, my sort of place.

I took the pebbled path around to Keats and Severn, already crying, sobbing hysterically—well, histrionically, then— and fell to my knees in the patch of ivy that fronted the graves. I hadn't cried so much since the madness of New Year's Day. I cried for all those who'd died too young, none of their promises kept, whose tombstones bore no name. These days everyone I knew seemed *writ in water*. Severn lay beside him,

the painter having lived into his eighty-fifth year, yet still remembered most for those fevered days and nights nearly sixty
years before.

TO THE MEMORY OF

JOSEPH SEVERN

DEVOTED FRIEND AND DEATH-BED COMPANION

OF

JOHN KEATS

WHOM HE LIVED TO SEE NUMBERED AMONG

THE IMMORTAL POETS OF ENGLAND

When I was sufficiently composed again I took my leave.
I'd had the place to myself for about a half hour, unless my
blubbering presence had simply scared off all the bachelor
schoolteachers come to pay their own homage. And by the
time I'd wandered back to Piazza Navona, gusts of smog swirling about me from the pitch of morning traffic, I was more
recovered from a lot of things than I understood at the time.
Craig was all packed and frantic lest we miss the train. I gave
him the barest outline of my visit to the Protestant Cemetery,
content to keep the histrionics to myself.

And when I returned to L.A. ten days later, my vigils at
3275 grew more and more intermittent. Not a conscious
thing, or indeed a happy turn of events. I'd finally shifted
ground, and knew at last that Roger wasn't there in Forest
Lawn at all. Or anywhere else. It would mostly now be a
journey for the sake of memory, the marking of his birthday
or his deathday or the anniversary of our meeting. A special
cortege if his parents or sister were in town, but that was only
once a year. I suppose I came to rely on the mail instead,
letters from readers of *Borrowed Time* to whom Roger was vividly alive, more alive than to me.

I met Stephen. Everyone said I'd moved on. After the
October action in Washington, and Stephen's arrest at the

FDA, we gave ourselves a few days' downtime in the Shenandoah Valley. We picnicked in the ruins of a brick plantation house, and later stumbled onto a Confederate graveyard. Buried where they'd fallen, it seemed, tombstones marking the end of soldiers who were only seventeen, some as young as fourteen. And may the gods forgive me, I'd passed once more into the realm of the picturesque. For this was as pretty a place as the old New England family plots fenced by iron staves, where I used to maunder away the afternoons of my adolescence.

Two months later, over New Year's on Kauai, we fulfilled a pledge to Adam Savage, Stephen's former roommate, who wanted his ashes scattered on a very specific beach. The northeast coast of the island, a dirt road winding down along the bank of a stream that was fed by a mountain rainforest—from deep in the interior where the rain never stopped. The stream debouched at Aliomanu Bay, an unmarked palmy strand where the sand was like powdered sugar. Picture-perfect.

We opened the box of ashes, difficult to scatter in the gusting breeze that white-capped the breakers. As Stephen poured the crushed bone into the maelstrom just where the fresh water met the salt, I intoned Edna Millay's "Dirge Without Music," trumpeting it into the wind. All in all an impressive ceremony, to us anyway, till we were confronted by a pair of natives carrying six-packs. "What're you guys dumping in that water?" one of them demanded, his anger barely suppressed. He had a hundred pounds on me.

"It's just a ritual," I replied pleasantly.

"Bullshit," his partner growled.

Stephen was done with the pouring, the last bits blown across the rippling current. We backed away to the car, smiling and nodding. They glared us out of there but made no move to attack. I understood the beach was theirs, no matter who held the deed. But I also knew in my own bones that they'd kill us for the trespass if they knew we'd dumped AIDS in the water. I thought back to them two years later, when my father told me a hospice had been denied a site in one of the Boston suburbs, because the townsfolk feared the runoff of rain from the roof would taint the groundwater with AIDS. This was before the fundamentalists began to picket AIDS funerals in the Midwest, mocking and spitting on the mourners.

My mother died the next winter, after what seemed a lifetime of struggling with emphysema. ("I know what it's like," she used to wheeze, "to have people treat you like your illness is all your own fault.") I flew into Boston in a blizzard, and was fishtailed the twenty miles north to Andover by an intrepid Sikh cabdriver. The funeral next morning, blue sky and a blinding snowscape, began with a service at Christ Episcopal. They opened the coffin one last time in the vestibule, so my father and brother and I could have a final something. I grazed her hand with my fingers, flinching from the icy cold, the waxen flesh. My father kissed her lips.

We buried her in the churchyard, in the snow behind the chancel—the gravediggers having huddled and decided the ground wasn't too frozen for the backhoe. My parents had acquired the plot the previous summer, proudly taking me there on my last visit home, so they could "show off the property." It was at the crest of a knoll, which fell in gentle terraces lush with the humid green of June, overlooking a hundred years of slate and granite markers in no particular ranks, faithful parishioners having settled in for the duration. Across on the next rise, separated by a country lane, was the Congregational graveyard, neighborly but a bit more trim, less shaggy than the Episcopal. You'd never believe you were fifty yards from the center of town.

"It's beautiful, isn't it?" declared my mother excitedly. "Daddy'll be able to come down and visit me and read his paper."

Beside the grave my father has set a small stone bench for

just that purpose. For six months after she died, I felt nothing. I'd tell my friends, "As soon as I have a feeling, I'll let you know." Not that the numbness wasn't a feeling, but it gave no access back to her.

It was sometime in early summer that I was driving with Stephen and his mother, riding in the back so they could talk. At one point he turned to her and asked, "Mom, do you need a place to visit?" We all knew what kind of place he meant. Dolores shook her head slowly: "No, it's not important to me."

I leaned forward and put in my two cents. "*I* need it," I said. And slick as a Bible salesman I made a pitch for Forest Lawn, the hill they called Revelation. We'd have to check to see if they allowed ashes to be buried up there, instead of in the safe-deposit boxes of the Columbarium. Otherwise the matter was settled, both of them leaving it up to me.

But it wasn't a detail we ever followed up on, the business of ashes in the ground. He got sick so unexpectedly on Labor Day, none of us really believing he was on his way out. Within ten days he was sealed in a mask, his lungs fed by a noisy oxygen push. He beckoned for paper and pen and scribbled these notes:

19/13/90

Cremated by After-Care (if possible) and if poss. *buried* (in the ground) close to you.

Would've wanted to convert to Living Trust but it seems a little late now, doesn't it?

Oh yes, later and later every hour. And the *déjà vu* a week later, riding five miles an hour at Forest Lawn with our Comfort Counselor, then abandoning the car for the steep walk up Revelation hill. Dolores and Ted, Stephen's father, paccompanied me, along with his sister Susan and Victor, our staunchest friend. I'd already determined to buy the highest plot of all, maybe fifteen feet above Roger, because our row was already filled. The family was pleased with the prospect and let me make the arrangements. There was in fact no problem about burying an urn of ashes in the ground.

"We usually sell these plots in pairs," purred the Counselor, thinking to make some room for me.

"Oh no, I'm going down there with Roger," I declared, pointing toward my own spot.

There was a beat of the purest confusion, as the Counselor tried to grapple with the meaning here. Slowly he began to put it together that I was widowed twice, a notion that clearly struck him as rather indelicate. Like that daft moment in *The Importance of Being Earnest,* when Jack's revelation that he's orphaned meets with the arch disapproval of Lady Bracknell:

> To lose one parent, Mr. Worthing, may be regarded
> as a misfortune; to lose both looks like carelessness.

And then Dolores stepped into the breach, turning to Victor to inquire, very no-nonsense: "Well, do *you* have a place?"

After a moment's left-footed dancing among us, we decided Victor would go beside Stephen. So we informed the Counselor that after all we would take the two-fer deal, which he duly recorded in his book of deeds, however questionable the arrangement seemed to him.

The funeral was three days later, with the burial after the service. I carried the porcelain urn, too small, it seemed, to hold all of him, for I was a connoisseur of ashes by now. Wondering if the remainder had been left in the oven, since the mortuary hadn't really liked us providing our own non-regulation urn, brought by Susan's Marine husband from his posting in Japan.

Numb again, number than even my mother had left me. The thing that sparked the tears was hearing from my friend Dan, who'd stood behind the scenes at the funeral to cue the music. Near him in the doorway lounged a pair of cemetery employees—polyester suits, not diggers—having a smoke. And trading fag jokes and AIDS jokes. Dan hissed at them to be quiet.

I reported them, of course, and of course they denied it. The Boss Comfort Counselor assured me over the phone that Forest Lawn had been the first to accept the dead of AIDS. In fact, she added smoothly, Forest Lawn was proud of having regular consciousness-raising sessions for all their employees, where the demonization of "all non-Christians" was rigorously discouraged. I thought I was going to puke if I didn't get off the phone fast.

I visited every day for a month, bringing with me a folder of pictures of Stephen—running through them like flash cards for a foreign tongue, except here they were wordless. My last jolt of rage had been spent ordering the bronze, on which I proposed to engrave:

STEPHEN F. KOLZAK

MY GUERRILLA, MY LOVE

1953–1990

DIED OF HOMOPHOBIA

DIED A HERO

BELOVED SON AND BROTHER

REAL ISN'T HOW YOU ARE MADE

YOU BECOME

It seemed the least I could give him by way of defiance, since he'd made it clear often enough that he wanted his body dumped on the White House lawn. The family protested as tactfully as it could. I excised *died of homophobia* and said I would have it on my grave instead. We retained the final quotation from *The Velveteen Rabbit*.

After a week or two I could cry a little, pricked by the weird juxtaposition of paying respects to Roger first, then the final climb to Stephen. Yet by the time Victor and I took off for Europe—a month to the day after burying Stevie—the pain had frozen over again. I'd hoped I might get through the grief weeping in cathedrals, but they pretty much left me cold. I even took Victor to the Protestant Cemetery in Rome, but Keats's grave had become just another story by then. More exalted than Forest Lawn, to be sure, where the Counselor had puffed with pride in the neighborhood, pointing out how close we were to Rick Nelson.

I think I've been to Revelation just three times in the last two years, in every case as an escort for one or the other family. The conversations on the hill are mostly suffused with memories—the good ones. In this the parents are wiser than I, who watch my body change and dwindle and seem able to recall only the suffering of the men I loved. These memories pursue me everywhere—on the radiation table, in the tunnel of an MRI, half my life in waiting rooms. I don't know where the certainty went, the solidity of the ground beneath me during the first year's visits to Roger. No matter what happened I'd end up here, the compass point of my journey's end. Surcease from the pain at last. Now that seems like another pretty story, no real comfort.

Last October Winston and I went to Paris, a city he'd never seen before. It was his idea to take the Metro out to Père-Lachaise, the permanent address for so many stellar Parisians. Mostly decrepit, not kept up, chockablock with phone-booth chapels whose stained-glass windows were kitsch to the max. Parisians being the least Catholic of Catholics, but with a sentimental streak a mile wide when it came to burying the dead.

They had just sandblasted Oscar Wilde, so the great Egyptian monument by Jacob Epstein—a Deco angel rampant, hovering in stone—was clean of all graffiti. No evidence of violence except the angel's privates, hacked away in the twenties and never replaced. Then Gertrude Stein, an unadorned slab with just her name and dates, very bourgeois. "But where's Alice?" I wondered aloud, thinking I'd misremembered their lying together. Then we walked around behind the slab through the unkempt ivy and found Alice's name in smaller letters, as if she'd averted her face from the spotlight one last time.

Around the next corner was Piaf's plot. Fortunately we had a map to find it, because she is listed first on the grave as Edith Giovanna Gassion (*dit* Piaf), her sparrow nickname consigned to parentheses. In any case it's a family plot, her own name no more prominent than the others. And we couldn't get too close, because she had a guardian attendant that day, a little man with a henna-rinsed rug and Poirot mustache who seemed profoundly offended by our presence. He was cleaning up the place, bearing away the withered floral tributes and dumping them in a *poubelle*. October tenth had been the twenty-ninth anniversary of her death, and people remembered still. Was this peculiar man, pushing seventy now, some member of the Gassion family? Or more likely one of the forty thousand mourners who broke through police barricades at the funeral, just to be closer to her.

The afternoon was sharp as an apple, clouds breaking up after days of rain, as we made our way around to the entrance again—one eye peeled for Proust and Isadora Duncan. We passed the line of memorials to those who'd died in the camps: Sachsenhausen, Buchenwald-Dora, Auschwitz, Ravensbruck, Mauthausen, each monument more horrorstruck than the last. Beseeching figures reaching their bony limbs to the sky, that the agony might lift. At the Mauthausen memorial there are

186 steps carved in the stone, to represent the Sisyphean task of the inmates, carrying rocks from the quarry—186 steps to reach level ground, only to be sent back for more rocks.[2]

We walked on somberly, mocked by the flashing sunlight through the chestnut trees, the necropolis having been washed clean by the rain. And then we entered a quarter that was overrun with graffiti, on every grave on every side. But not the urban graffiti we were used to, the hieratic mock-Cyrillic of the spray can. Here the notes and tributes were rather more formal: SEX DRUGS AND ROCK 'N' ROLL; WE LOVE YOU, JIM; THE MUSIC NEVER DIES. Intensifying in volume as we neared the grave itself, scarcely a bare spot left on the bourgeois marble—useless to sandblast such a torrent.

At Morrison's place was a curious assembly of punk Eurokids and retro American hippies, sitting about and smoking but altogether subdued and respectful. Hard to tell the difference, frankly, between this ragtag troupe and the fussy man with the henna job, as far as the fervor of memory went. There's no one way to visit such places, no prescribed amount of tears. But always it seems we make the journey to enter a river of memory larger than our poor tributaries, the brooks of spring that have dried up by summer's end.

Inevitably, Père-Lachaise is defined by its most distinguished residents, so many and so varied that one cannot help but move through its alleys like a tourist. As long as you're there you might as well check out Proust. No disrespect in that, but hardly the level of pilgrimage that brings you to Kiowa Ranch or the Protestant Cemetery.

My own touchstone in Paris lies at the center of the city— the hub of France, in fact, from which all distances and road

---

2. For an *aide-memoire* to Père-Lachaise, I am indebted to the superb guide to the cemeteries of Paris by Judi Culbertson and Tom Randall, *Permanent Parisians* (Chelsea, Vt.: Chelsea Green Publishing Co., 1986).

signs take their measure. If you are a hundred kilometers from Paris, it means you are just so far from the west portal of Notre Dame. At the stern tip of the Ile de la Cité, just behind the brawny cathedral, lies the monument to the French deported to the camps. It's barely identified, easy to miss, a gated garden in front of what looks like a fortress wall. On either side a pair of steep stairways lead down to a walled courtyard at the level of the river.

A concrete holding pen, it feels like, with a single opening onto the river, a barred gate like a portcullis. You are meant to feel that here is where they will board you under guard, onto prison ships that will carry you to your doom. If you turn away you're confronted by the narrow entrance that pierces the fortress wall and beckons you into a kind of cave.

The first thing you see, directly in front of you, is a dim-lit tunnel receding deep under the island. The tunnel is paved with tiny glass beads of light, one for each of the two hundred thousand deportees. On the end wall of the tunnel is a bright light, almost a searchlight, which I've been told is intended to represent hope. But it's hard not to see it as the beam of a train, bearing down on all of us. At your feet there's a sort of bronze sarcophagus, containing the remains of an *inconnu,* an unknown inmate.

You are not permitted to enter the tunnel, only to wander around the vestibule. On the walls are carved quotations from the writers of the Resistance—Sartre, Camus, St. Exupéry, Vercors. But the carver's alphabet is jagged, as if every letter had been etched in the stone with a sharpened spoon handle. Defacement of a very high order, the graffiti of the damned. Curiously uplifting in its way, because there isn't a false step anywhere, no Disney simplification, no tidying up. As you walk out into daylight again, incised above the doorway in the same prisoner's alphabet is the final admonition: FORGIVE BUT DON'T FORGET.

I wasn't numb there at all. No tears exactly, but a sense in which I was centered by my grief. All my dead around me, bearing me up. We were in Paris seven days, staying in a small hotel on the Ile Saint Louis, barely a hundred yards from the monument. I paid a visit every day and usually had the place to myself. Like some version of the man with the henna wig, I grew quite proprietary, gladly offering simultaneous translations of the words in the stone to American tourists struggling with their high school French. One afternoon I was joined by an old man who told me he had survived two years at Bergen-Belsen. After a half-hour of showing *me* the monument, I wasn't sure whether he'd be offended if I offered him a gratuity. When I did, he accepted it heartily and gave me a bear hug, then took off to have himself a glass.

All of which somehow leads me back to 3275. I will probably die without forgiving anyone, certainly not the *Kapos* and the Commandants of Reagan/Bush and their genocidal politics of AIDS. It's been engraved too long on my brain that my epitaph should proclaim—

DIED OF HOMOPHOBIA

MURDERED BY HIS GOVERNMENT

Still room of course for a line or two of uplift, a scrap of Shakespeare, but I haven't settled on that yet. My heart is too exhausted to sustain the bitterness anymore, not even against the calumnies of my enemies. The writer who trashed me twelve years ago in the *Native* has kept up his campaign. "It isn't even English," he remarked to an interviewer last summer, shuddering at my prose. He has a friend who calls him, he says, and reads whole paragraphs of me, reducing them both to whinnies of laughter.

But his malice has lost its power to make me feel *writ in water*. AIDS has taught me precisely what I'm writ in, blood and bone and viral load. I can't tell anymore whom I am addressing with my epitaph. The accidental tourist? Or my own grieving friends who can't even parse their losses anymore, who don't need bronze to recall me. And after all, I've been visiting my own grave for years now—*pre-need,* as they call it at Forest Lawn—and I don't require any further vigil from anybody.

Unless it is some kind of safety zone. And as long as there's no piety in the gesture. I don't like flowers, but the deer do. Keats and Lawrence and Stevenson all died of their lungs, robbed by a century whose major products were soot and sulfur. We queers on Revelation hill, tucking our skirts about us so as not to touch our Mormon neighbors, died of the greed of power, because we were expendable. If you mean to visit any of us, it had better be to make you strong to fight that power. Take your languor and easy tears somewhere else. Above all, don't pretty us up. Tell yourself: *None of this ever had to happen.* And then go make it stop, with whatever breath you have left. Grief is a sword, or it is nothing.

THE POLITICS
OF SILENCE

THIS MORNING in *The Washington Post* there happened to be a pairing of my picture with Pat Buchanan's picture. I'm sure I'm the only one who noticed that the pictures were printed askew, so that the bottom part of mine lapped over his—almost as if I'm trying to butt in front of him. Which I am, as a matter of fact. But think of the jowl-flapping and the wounded bluster at Pat's house this morning, at such an egregious example of *lèse-majesté*. Not to worry, Pat. I'll see to it that they don't link us romantically, even in the tabloids. We're both married men, after all, doing our leatherneck best to uphold family.

The reporter in the *Post* also notes that this could be one of my last public appearances, which is a pretty cheap way to fill a house. Have no fear. I do not expect to keel over in the next forty-five minutes. But I am reminded of a story.

These remarks—in slightly shaggier form—were delivered in a public forum at the Library of Congress, on 28 January 1993, as part of the celebration of National Book Week.

My friend Bruce Vilanch is the primo comic writer in Los Angeles, the master of the one-liner, who's written material for some of the funniest people in the world. Not long ago he wrote a Vegas show for Jim Bailey, the incomparable female illusionist. Bruce flew up to Vegas for opening night, and they'd saved him a nice ringside table. This was one of those evenings where Jim wasn't going to impersonate several ladies, but just Judy Garland.

The orchestra struck up a fanfare, and Jim came strutting out dressed as Judy, belting "Swanee." Bruce is sitting next to a couple from the Midwest, so encased in polyester they were fireproof. And the man turns to his wife and says, in some bewilderment, "I thought she was dead."

And his wife kind of pats his knee and replies with a knowing smile: "It's the daughter."

That's what I think of when people write to my publisher asking, "Is Paul Monette still alive?" No, but the daughter is.

I have titled these remarks "The Politics of Silence." A friend of mine suggested to me last week that *Becoming a Man* would have been a better book without the diatribe of the first five pages. A more seasoned writer, he seemed to imply, would have tossed those pages out before submitting the book for publication. We talked at some length about whether art should be political or not. His own sister is a novelist, a very fine one, and it was she who'd heaved my book across the room after feeling assaulted by those five pages.

I said to my friend: "Is your sister political?"

And he replied: "No, she's an artist."

This is not something I can agree to anymore. It is simply not enough to be an artist, unengaged. If you live in political times, if the lightning rod of history quivers with fire on your roof, then all art is political. And all art that is not *consciously* so partakes of the messiness of politics, if only to flee it. People still went to the opera in Nazi Germany. People still read books that were pleasant and diverting.

Robin Lane Fox, a massively learned historian of religion, says most people believe that the Christian world was a fait accompli, a historical inevitability. But in point of fact, until Constantine converted to Christianity in 313, the western world was a battleground between pagans and Christians. The pagans were an urban, sophisticated class—not unlike us. They had their mysteries, and of course they had their gods, very human gods. So one of the first things the early popes did was systematically destroy the pagan texts, or lock them up in monasteries. Professor Fox was only able to reconstruct a semblance of the pagan world by going through ancient cemeteries reading the gravestones.

If you destroy the record, you destroy the truth.

I've learned in my adult life that the will to silence the truth is always and everywhere as strong as the truth itself. So it is a necessary fight we will always be in: those of us who struggle to understand our common truths, and those who try to erase them. The first Nazi book burning, I would have you remember, was of a gay and lesbian archive.

In that light, I think there could not be a more appropriate place to talk about censorship than the Library of Congress. Censorship is such a subtle thing. Most of it we don't even hear about, because it's done in the dark by dirty and ashamed people, by self-appointed judges who are convinced they know what's best for all of us. These are the people who always keep a match ready to start a conflagration.

We must not be lulled into a false sense of security by our First Amendment freedoms, freedoms which have never in the history of this nation been under so much attack. It is a wholly specious argument to say we are engaged in a fight between literary standards and moral standards. These matters are very specific and very concrete—the withholding of a particular book from the library shelf, the capitulation to pressure that would bar from the hungering reader books as diverse as *The*

Wizard of Oz, Huckleberry Finn, and *The Catcher in the Rye.* Not to mention *The Origin of Species.*

Just this week we've been struggling with the very nub of this issue. My colleague Dorothy Allison, who was nominated for a National Book Award in fiction for an exquisite and remarkable novel called *Bastard out of Carolina,* was abruptly canceled from giving a National Book Week speech in Oklahoma. And the most tragic thing about it is that they made their decision to censor without ever having seen the book, let alone read it. They just heard through their own grapevine that Dorothy is a lesbian poet, and suddenly it was deemed inappropriate that she address an audience that might include children.

There has been endless backing and filling and covering of tracks over this incident, with every Oklahoma library official bending backward to assure us it was all just an innocent glitch of scheduling. The schedule, you see, had been set in stone months before, and there simply wasn't room for any more authors. Really? One wonders if they would have found room for Toni Morrison or John Updike.[1]

For forty-five years, since the end of the war, there has been a campaign to tell people that Anne Frank never existed, that her *Diary* was a pernicious fiction, foisted on the public by the Jewish conspiracy. They haven't won yet, the rewriters of history. Anne Frank's book is still there, in every library.

---

1. After much brouhaha—during which the text of this speech was considered unacceptable to be published as a pamphlet by the Library of Congress because of my remarks on the Dorothy Allison affair—a compromise was finally reached. All parties agreed to the following footnote: *The Center for the Book in the Library of Congress and the Oklahoma Department of Libraries strongly disagree with Mr. Monette's interpretation of the Dorothy Allison Incident.* In the circumstances, it seems more than a little ironic that an attempt was made to censor a speech on censorship. Meanwhile, I am not expecting any flood of invitations to speak to the good people of Oklahoma.

Teenagers still get to read it. But a lot of fundamentalists don't want it in schools, because it's "obscene." And while they're at it, they don't want the Holocaust taught either, because it never happened.

Now their tactic is to check out offending books from the library and throw them away. Such has been the fate of *Heather Has Two Mommies* and *Daddy's Roommate,* both published by Alyson Press in Boston. Sasha Alyson has publicly declared that he will send these books out free to any library that wants them, but within a week they've usually vanished.

I want to say that it's difficult to speak of my fellow citizens as my enemies. I never expected to grow up with enemies. But then, I never expected to get this far as a man, or to become so involved in the politics of my time. It's clear now that the fundamentalists' agenda of lies and hate grows daily, and it's Protestant and it's Catholic and it's Muslim and it's Jewish. It starts as a kind of lunatic fringe in each religion, till the fringe consumes the center.

It's no secret that I'm very hard on the Pope, a figure of consummate evil and irresponsibility. A lot of people take umbrage at those remarks, saying, "You really shouldn't be criticizing other people's faith—we still have freedom of religion in this country." Unfortunately, I think what's happened to our freedom of religion is that we're free to be nutcake fundamentalist Christians and hate everybody else. Meanwhile, no one seems capable of drawing the line between freedom of religion and the naked politics of hate.

I have great respect for anyone's relationship to his or her God, just as I have enormous esteem for priests and sisters I know who constitute a kind of resistance movement in the Church. These are the ones who believe in Liberation Theology. These are the nuns who have come out pro-choice, unleashing a witch hunt against them by the Vatican. They deserve our support and gratitude.

And as for their leaders and commandants, I've always

been suspicious of their obsessive interest in other people's sex lives. People who spend all their time combatting the sexuality of others suffer from a kind of sexual-compulsive personality disorder. And it's they who give tacit approval for the violence against us, whether it's a bunch of drunken louts who attack us in the streets with baseball bats, or the systematic wrecking of gay kids' lives by fundamentalist parents. Many of these so-called leaders, of course, are homosexuals who can't come to terms with themselves, and they displace their own guilt and discomfort on us.

One of the most chilling things I had to write in my auto-biography was that I told homophobic jokes when I was in the closet, anything to cover my own tracks. It's hard to find a corrective role model, because there really isn't a gay or lesbian spokesperson in Punditland. So many of these strutting opin-ion-makers—like Buchanan and Will, James Kilpatrick and William F. Buckley—have been good little Catholic boys all their lives. They were taught their intolerance in the Church of the forties and fifties, and apparently they have rigorously avoided contact with us sodomites and heathens ever since, so as not to contaminate their self-righteousness. Their fathers and their priests also believed that the Jews murdered Their Lord, but that one's been relegated to a back burner, too controver-sial after the Holocaust.

I would like to draw a distinction, though, between ho-mophobia and homo-ignorance. There's much more homo-ignorance than homophobia, I think. And though it's difficult for us as a people, as a tribe, to hear the hate spewed at us, we know it's better for that hatred to be public than for it to be secret. When I speak of the politics of silence, I don't just speak of the silence of gay and lesbian people for fifteen hun-dred years—those rare exceptions like Whitman or Michel-angelo notwithstanding. I want you to understand that that silence is as much self-imposed as imposed by our enemies. We learn the message of their hatred all too well, and we choose the closet, hoping to protect ourselves. And that very invisibility is just what our enemies want, the silence that stunts our self-esteem.

Sometimes I think that the ones who hate us can't stand the fact that we've won out over oppression. They can't stand to see us leading happy and productive lives. A joyful gay or lesbian person messes with their minds profoundly. I always tell parents who are in pain after discovering their sons and daughters are gay—It's not my fault, they say; I know it's genetic, but I don't want my kid to live a pariah's life—I tell them life is difficult for everyone. The struggle for true openness and intimacy is a lifelong struggle for all of us, gay and straight alike. And besides, a difficult life brings you to the core of yourself, where you learn what justice is and how it has to be fought for. Despite all the hate and intolerance—at fever pitch these days—I would not give up a minute of the last seventeen years of being out. I'm myself now, not somebody else. I've had a full and joyous life, and that even includes the decade of AIDS. I am able to be as angry as I am at our government's indifference, as despairing as I am about how far away a cure is, and still be a happy man, because I'm so glad to be out. And because I've learned that anger against injustice is good for you. It sharpens your soul.

I consider the work I've been doing in the last six years as a kind of letter to my gay and lesbian children in the future, to them and their allies. We need our straight allies more than ever. Most of our families do the best they can to bring us up whole and make us worthy citizens. But it's a very rare person who manages to arrive at adulthood without being saddled by some form of racism or sexism or homophobia. It is our task as grownups to face those prejudices in ourselves and rethink them. The absolute minimum we can get out of such a self-examination is tolerance, one for another. We gay and lesbian people believe we should be allowed to celebrate ourselves and give back to the larger culture, make our unique contributions—but if all we can get is tolerance, we'll take it. And build on it.

We don't know what history is going to say even about this week, or where the gay and lesbian revolution is going to go. But we are a revolution that has come to be based very, very strongly on diversity. We have to fight like everyone else to be open to that diversity; but I love Urvashi Vaid's idea that it's not a matter of there being one of each on every board and every faculty and every organization. It's a matter of being *each in one*. You'll pardon my French, but it's not so hard to be politically correct. All you have to do is not be an asshole.

I want to say something about Primo Levi and implicitly about Anne Frank. For me they are the two greatest writers about the Holocaust. Primo Levi was an Italian chemist who was in Auschwitz for a long, long time. After he was liberated, he wrote about the camps for the next forty years, one book after another. The first of these is brilliant, and you wouldn't have thought he needed to do it again. But he was so convinced that history would try to lie about his experience that he had to keep writing about it to make sure he kept up with his own truth.

By the mid-fifties, commandants from the camps were beginning to publish their memoirs. "My camp wasn't like that," they said. "We had a very good arts and crafts program at my camp." All this surreal rethinking of history, the art of erasure—and Levi would not have that. He had too much moral force as a writer, a kind of moral fiber that I also associate with Elie Wiesel, who could face President Reagan and declare: "Mr. President, you do not belong at Bitburg. I have seen with my own eyes children thrown in the ovens. Bitburg is not your place. Your place is with the survivors, not with the SS troops."

As I remember, the White House handled that moral

dilemma by making sure that when they got to Bitburg, as scheduled, everyone turned his back on the SS graves. Not a very noble or courageous statement, I'm afraid.

I repeat, the first order of business of people who would obliterate the truth is to get the books. It's all so precious and fragile. Aristotle's books wound up in the great library at Ephesus in Asia Minor, of which nothing is left but an eloquent and towering facade. What happened to Aristotle's books is that Antony stole them. He sacked the library at Ephesus and brought the books to Alexandria as a tribute to Cleopatra. And you all know the rest of the story—the library at Alexandria burned, a conflagration of papyrus and waxen tablets. So we don't have a scrap of Aristotle's personal library anymore.

All so precious and fragile. The only reason we have Sappho's poems is that a copy on papyrus was rolled up and plugged in a wine jug. The jug was stored in a cave, and by the time it was found—millennia later—there was just the neck of the jug left, with this peculiar stopper still in place. People knew enough about Sappho's writing from other sources to realize what they'd found. The blanks in Sappho's text are where the acid of the wine ate into the papyrus.

I wear a button that says I AM SALMAN RUSHDIE. I've been wearing it off and on at literary events, ever since the *fatwa* was first declared against him. He's apparently not an easy man. It's definitely not an easy book, if any of you have actually read *The Satanic Verses*. But it's so clearly art, so clearly rich in irony—but mullahs don't understand that. Rushdie has spoken fiercely and eloquently all around the world, saying, "You're *all* me, you know. If you let me go down, let me get murdered, then you're murdered too."

He's still trying to get some governments to contact Iran and use their clout to get this thing rescinded. Canada has finally agreed to speak for him. And when he came to Washington? Well, that brilliant philosopher, Marlin Fitzwater, declared, "Rushdie? No, he's not coming to the White House. To us he's just another author on a book tour."

We will have no test for freedom of speech if the passion for it atrophies. If we are content with sound bites and TV bullshit, there will be no words to stir our hearts or even to tell us what our hearts are for. The outsider always knows that, and gay and lesbian people have always been outsiders. And always ready to fight. For a year we battled the National Endowment for the Arts, to keep it free from political manipulation.

Were I in the President's position, I don't know that I would have gone forward with the lifting of the military ban as quickly as he did. To me AIDS was the more crucial emergency that needed to be addressed. But it turns out not to matter, since either issue engages the virulence of the right wing, that frightening need to dance on our graves. The step they're going to take is to stop asking recruits, "Are you a homosexual?" Frankly, what they really need to ask is, "Are you homophobic?" Then they would know who needed some serious counseling.

I think everybody's teachable. But that is why the most pernicious of the right-wing "compromises" is to say we won't be asked our sexual orientation, but we mustn't *talk* about it either. Once again, the silence that equals death. We've had ten years of a witch hunt, instituted by Reagan, and three hundred million dollars spent ridding the services of gay and lesbian people. *That's* the crime.

As we reclaim our history, we don't seek to exclude anybody. There's a turmoil now among certain scholars to punish great books from the past for not having the right attitude about gay and lesbian. Yet those books saved my life, even though none of the classics I read growing up ever spoke my name. Despite that, their greatness as literature had something to speak to my heart.

We needn't tar the past for the sake of the present. As

long as we understand that there's no excuse *anymore*. One of the great breakthroughs I made as a writer in the last ten years was to be able to write about lesbians. Ten years ago I silenced myself because I was so afraid I would get it wrong and come out with a stupid stereotype that wouldn't help anybody. It was my friend Katherine Forrest who said to me, "We have to populate our books with one another."

Sometimes I say to myself, "My God, we're the freest gay and lesbian people in the world." That's a stunning realization in a country where people murder us at will and pass slavery laws against us. But I have an inkling of how bad the situation is in the third world and the fourth world. In some Muslim countries people are put to death for homosexual "behavior."

We are the crucial issue of the nineties, no doubt about *that*. We are the crucible in which it will be decided whether or not we can all come together as a people. The pie is going to get smaller and smaller, and people are going to turn more and more toward demagogues and religious crazies. *We* are the Salman Rushdies of our age. If we go down, then you all go down.

So many people have written to me since I published *Becoming a Man*. The book has a life of its own; it's more real than I am. People expect me to be as wise as *it* is, and I'm not. But so many have said it echoes their own story, women and men both, and everyone seems to conclude the same thing. We *must* be the last generation to suffer this stunted growing. We must somehow reach out to all our troubled brothers and sisters, reach out to their families, and stop the prejudice now.

There was a great recoil in this country from the tactics and language of the 1992 Republican convention. (I preferred it in the original German, as Molly Ivins acidly put it.) We are in the middle of Pat Buchanan's holy war, whether we like it or not. He and his co-religionists have a real vision of slaughtering their enemies, a regular jihad. They don't seem to understand that the Bible doesn't give them or anyone else the right to pass judgment on how a person loves.

Two can play that game, you know. Any number of scholars have read those subhuman passages from Leviticus, and they've gone back to the Aramaic, explaining over and over again that this bigotry involves a staggering amount of mistranslation. If you went with all the strictures in Leviticus, we'd all be standing on our heads in sheep dung.

For me, Jesus is patently queer. And I don't mean that as an insult to him. I'm speaking of his role as a shaman and as a healer and as a prophet. Besides, his hair is a little too well coifed, if you know what I mean. So don't throw that book in my face, because that book doesn't belong to anyone.

I get a lot of credit—poster child credit—for being a writer with AIDS who manages to get through a lecture without keeling over. I don't know if AIDS has made me so brave as a writer. I don't know whether it has widened my heart the way witnessing the world at war widened Anne Frank's heart. Who would have thought that the greatest account of that war, the one that would sear the hearts of the future, would be written by a fourteen-year-old girl? And a fourteen-year-old who went to her death believing that people were fundamentally good. That's where I fail, much of the time.

In the thirties, Picasso was asked: "What if they took everything away from you? All your paints and all your brushes and all your canvases. What would you do then? What if they put you in prison with nothing—no chalk, no nothing?"

And he said without a moment's pause: "I'd draw with my spit on the prison walls."

The winner of last year's Nobel Peace Prize, a woman named Daw Aung San Suu Kyi, has been under house arrest in Burma for years now. She went back to Burma to take care of her ailing mother. She was a free woman, married to an Oxford don. But her father was the founder of modern Burma, and when the generals took over they told her she wasn't allowed to stay and care for her mother. They wanted her *out,* so they could continue the repression and destruction of the society without any witnesses. And she said no, she wouldn't go.

She's gravely ill now from a hunger strike, and she's told the generals that she'll gladly leave. But she said, "I want all political prisoners released, and I want to walk to the airport." It's twenty miles from her prison house to the airport. And she has so rallied the spirit of her people that the generals rightly fear that the whole country would turn out to cheer her if she took that twenty-mile walk. So please think about her when you think of the politics of silence.

Or think of the Russian poet Irina Ratushinskaya. When she was in the labor camps she would write her poems on a bar of soap with a burnt matchstick. She would write a line in the soap and memorize it; and when she was sure she would never forget it, she would wash it away and go on to the next line.

The difference between having freedom as a writer and having no freedom is as narrow as the choice that the truth is important. In speech after speech Rushdie says: "What do you want a writer to be? How much will you stand up for what a writer says?"

I had one great teacher in high school, the man who more than anyone made it possible for me to write. His name was Dudley Fitts; and oh, he was such a brilliant man. He had translated the edition of Sophocles we read in senior English. He would sit in front of the class and read it in Greek while we followed along in English, and it was like being transported back to the ancient world.

He spent a lot of time on Antigone's dilemma. If you re-member, Antigone buries her brother, collecting his body from the field of battle despite the edict of Creon the king, that she will be put to death if she does so. That is the great choice in classical literature between law and conscience. Antigone chose conscience and thus chose her fate.

"O tomb, O marriage chamber," she says as she goes to her death. And the Chorus comes out to comment on what it all means. (Garry Wills could say this so much better than I.) "Isn't man wonderful?" sings the Chorus. "He longed so much to speak his heart that he taught himself language, so that what was inside him could be spoken to the world."

I was given my heart back when I came out. People say I'm too hard on myself, but if you were to read the dreary poems I wrote in my twenties, you would discover they're about nothing because they're not about me. They are not the truth.

So I guess what I would say to my gay and lesbian brothers and sisters, especially to the gay and lesbian children of the next generation, and to all our friends and allies, is: Come out when you can. I know it's not easy for everybody. People misguidedly try to protect their families, or they're rightfully afraid of the impact on their jobs. I have fortunately been in a position to be way, way out on both issues—being a gay man and having AIDS.

In the meantime, even if you must keep your own life secret, hold on and support us. My friend Betty Berzon, a psychologist, says it's not enough to come out. Coming out is just the first step, a kind of outer coming out. Then we have to begin the inner coming out, looking to nourish our own battered self-esteem.

To really be a gay and lesbian citizen, you have to also give back to your community. You have to reach out and help it. Some of the people who hate us so much think we're out to indoctrinate their children. Frankly, we're trying to save their children from suicide. A third of all teen suicides are gay and lesbian, and they're all unnecessary, and we want those kids to have a chance.

To them, I try to get across the message that they're not alone.

I'll close with a thought that's been terribly important to me lately, about "The Star-Spangled Banner." Always, you understand, the right wing questions our patriotism, as if the flag were all theirs as well as the Bible. In light of which, there's a wonderful remark Kurt Vonnegut made in one of his novels, which I quoted when I won this award in November. He says "The Star-Spangled Banner" is the only national anthem in the world that ends with a question:

> Oh, say, does that star-spangled banner yet wave
> O'er the land of the free and the home of the brave?

The speaker of those words, I've always thought, is a wounded soldier who's only been able to see the flag during the long night of fighting by the glare of the rockets. And yet I also see the speaker as a refugee, clinging to his place on these shores, or just dreaming of freedom in a far-off country from which he longs to emigrate.

It makes me immensely proud as a free American that Kathleen Battle was able to sing "We Shall Overcome" on the very spot where Marian Anderson sang because the DAR threw her out of Constitution Hall. All of it under the gaze of Lincoln, who prayed that we would be worthy of the "angels of our better natures." We all stand taller because we were here on the same planet with a man as great as Justice Marshall, buried today.

I came to Washington in 1975, wide-eyed. Roger was able to get us into the Supreme Court to hear them argue the death penalty. I was an amateur student of the Court at the time, and it was stunning to sit in the audience and see Hugo Black and William O. Douglas and Thurgood Marshall and William Brennan and Lewis Powell and Harry Blackmun, right there in the flesh. Robert Bork was arguing for the government, as solicitor-general. Anthony Amsterdam was defense counsel, defending three black men who'd shot up a convenience store in the South. And the curious thing that I felt, watching them all day long, was that I never once thought about who was a conservative and who was a liberal. It never crossed my mind. I thought I was in the presence of philosopher-kings.

All so precious and fragile. Don't let anyone tell you that the truth can't disappear. If I believe in anything, rather than God, it's that I am part of something that goes all the way back to Antigone, and that whatever speaks the truth of our hearts can only make us stronger. Can only give us the power to counter the hate and bigotry and heal this addled world.

Just remember: You are not alone.

MUSTERING

WE DIDN'T KNOW till the last minute whether we'd make it to Washington for the March. I couldn't pack; I couldn't even think. In those last days I was on a scavenger hunt for medicine, a doctor who would somehow halt the downward slide. I was just coming off four weeks of radiation—my second course of it in three months, only this time it hadn't worked. My radiation team had triumphed in the first go-round, excising a cluster of KS lesions on my penis, more horrible to contemplate than causing any pain or problems making water. Radiation hadn't even hurt. That is, until the radiation burn came on at the end of treatment. Two weeks of walking bow-legged as a cowboy, wearing boxer shorts sized XXL so as not to rub myself the wrong way.

But this second course was a trickier business. The area to be zapped was my left thigh, which had been swelling with edema for some months now, returning to "normal" size only after a night spent prone in bed. No pain. You couldn't *see* anything—no purple spots, I mean—and for months my oncologist's advice was to leave it alone. The thigh hadn't really "bloomed" yet, and Dr. Thommes wanted to keep me off chemo as long as possible. This is called buying time in the cancer business. Besides, I had a slot in a protocol at UCLA for a new drug that showed promise in treating KS, and I'd have to drop out of the study if I was taking chemo. The problem was, the UCLA drug still wasn't available—a monthly broken promise by the pharmaceutical company, which kept finding reasons to postpone the study. My swollen leg did not factor into their decisions.

All my oncology team agreed I'd better go ahead with more radiation, for the area along my inner thigh had begun to harden—turning "woody," to use their grisly euphemism. Clearly the KS had spread to my lymph system. Still, I plunged ahead confidently, stoked at having been given back my penis minus the purple nasties, convinced my thigh would respond as quickly.

But two weeks into treatment the leg was swelling more, not less. Blips of lesions began to bloom on the surface of the radiated skin. The most difficult aspect of all of this—getting over to the hospital every day, finding a parking space without resorting to my Uzi—had finally become a physical challenge. I'd developed the beginnings of a gimp as I struggled to get out of the car and made the trek to Radiology.

They finally gave up on my thigh, muttering in frustration about this "leg thing." It was cropping up more and more these days, it seemed, and dodging the zap of their x-rays. I could've told them that my very first case of AIDS—César in 1983—had started with a leg like mine, swelling over the next two years till it was truly the size of a tree trunk, woody indeed. Then it began to suppurate and developed gangrene, not perhaps the thing that took him in the end but the major assault of his illness. I *knew* about this thing. But since it was time to move on to chemo, I blocked all memories of the sufferings of the past. Surely treatment had advanced in the ten years since César had been experimented on.

What it all had to do with Washington was that my first dose of chemo was scheduled for Tuesday, the 20th of April, the day before we were leaving for the March. *Don't worry,* the chemo team reassured me, *we can take care of this.* Sounding ominously like the radiation team a month before, though it seemed bad faith to bring that up now. Perversely, now, I missed the radiation staff—missed even the daily trips to Century City Hospital. As if to leave behind the brute technology of zapping were to wave goodbye to a simpler world, Arcadian compared to the exigencies of chemo.

Still, they all agreed I could go to Washington as planned, though warning me I wouldn't be at my best for a few days after. Meanwhile they would withhold the *really* toxic drug in the chemo arsenal, the one that takes your hair and makes you want to throw up all the time. For that they would wait till we got home. Despite these assurances, Winston and I were gun-shy. The previous June, just hours before we were to leave on a book tour, the bags packed, my doctor called and ordered me into the hospital. My brain scan had revealed that I was abloom with toxoplasmosis (I was turning into a veritable garden of exotic flowers), thus explaining my peculiar site-specific headaches, as if I'd been beaned by a golf ball. There followed the arduous hit-and-miss of trying to find a treatment I wasn't allergic to. We stopped the infection with 566C80, a last-ditch protocol. My brain had been stable for seven months, but the memory of unpacking lingered, a curse on flying away.

And now the headaches had returned. The doctors deemed it prudent that I submit to another brain scan. Which I did on the Monday before the Wednesday departure. I was scarcely able to keep the two emergencies separate in my head, the brain infection and the cancer—it was like careening down a mountain road and having to steer two cars at once.

Why were we going to Washington? Our friend Victor put it most succinctly: "I guess because we're still here."

On Tuesday evening when I came home from a string of

doctors' appointments, Winston had everything out, ready to go in the suitcases. My barber kindly paid a house call, hacking at my unruly mop so I would be presentable in the nation's capital, instead of looking like the fourth Stooge. I dripped my daily IV infusion to keep from going blind. By midnight the phone hadn't rung, so Winston went ahead and packed the cases. We hardly slept at all, expecting a six-thirty cab to the airport. I slipped a volume of Sappho's poems into my carry-on bag, and we headed out.

Late at night, never asleep before three, I'd taken to reading the fragments of her poems to settle myself—a respite from the brain-and-cancer obstacle course. It was Winston who'd come across one of the lyrics in his reading:

> Without warning
>
> As a whirlwind
> swoops on an oak
> Love shakes my heart.

I dug out my Mary Barnard translation so he could see the full range, finding myself captivated all over again. One night I looked Sappho up in the *Oxford Companion,* reading aloud the citation, Winston beside me in bed. I read the part about her being "the leading personality among a circle of women and girls who must have comprised her audience." The great poet of Lesbos, who made the island synonymous with women loving women. The entry ends with a judgment, almost casual in its certainty:

> Sappho created a form of subjective lyric never equaled in the ancient world in its immediacy and intensity.[1]

---

1. M. C. Howatson, ed., *The Oxford Companion to Classical Literature* (Oxford, 1990), pages 506–507.

Dazzling, that. I turned to Winston and said, *Do you know how good you have to be to be called unequaled after twenty-six hundred years?* I felt just then an enormous pride of ancestry, and a vivid sense of linkage with the language of the heart.

> Some say a cavalry corps
> some infantry, some, again,
> will maintain that the swift oars
>
> of our fleet are the finest
> sight on dark earth; but I say
> that whatever one loves, is.

On the plane to D.C., fully half the passengers queer, I leafed through *Vanity Fair* and *The Advocate* and the L.A. *Times,* but turned again to Sappho. Caught up in her un-equaled feeling, I was overcome with a great relief. Even if all the books are burned, I thought, somehow the emotions sur-vive. Twenty-six hundred years from now, someone will still be struggling to set it all down—perhaps without any sense of ancestry, but that won't really matter. The grope for immedi-acy and intensity continues.

I understand that this is a somewhat discredited view of the classics, too romantic by half, the appropriation of classical sources and the certainty that we moderns feel just like they did, or they like us. A distinctly nineteenth-century notion, akin to the sloppy idea that we experience Democracy on a sort of continuum with Athens in the Golden Age, ignoring their slaves and the general powerlessness of women. Add to this the headache-making rift in gay and lesbian studies, where the "social constructionists" (also called "new-inventionists") argue that there was no such thing as a gay or lesbian person until late in the nineteenth century, when "homosexual" was coined. Plato would never have thought of himself as gay, nor would Sappho or anyone else, because the world was perceived entirely differently. The post-structural theorists define what "knowing" is, and it doesn't include self-knowledge about sexual orientation.

Doesn't make any sense to me, but then my own limited expertise is the history of the heart, and there are no breaks in its utterance through all written time. What else do you do with a lyric like this:

Afraid of losing you

I ran fluttering
like a little girl
after her mother.[2]

Self-awareness so deep it takes the breath away, whether or not the poet would ever have said she was a lesbian. (As opposed to Lesbian, which she surely was, as a resident of that deep-harbored island off the coast of Asia Minor.) I guess I have to accept that I read with a nineteenth-century eye, while secretly hoping for the passing of new-inventionism.

In addition to which, there had just been published in the previous week a study which averred that gay people are only one percent of the population, thus starting a new firestorm of marginalization among the Christian right. A study that turned out to be checkered from beginning to end. Only men were interviewed, for one thing, and some of us were beginning to feel that queer didn't parse that way, separating by gender. We were gender-*variant* if anything. And if not yet a fully unified tribe, then at least groping toward it. In addition, as Dr. Betty Berzon remarked, all the questions in the study were about sexual activity. "If you never had sex again for the next forty

---

2. All quotations from Sappho are from Mary Barnard's *Sappho: A New Translation* (Univ. of California Press, 1966).

years," she told me, "you'd still be gay." But perhaps most tellingly, thirty percent of the men contacted by the researchers refused to take part in a sexual survey. The interviews were face to face, the interviewer always a woman, and there was no perception that closeted men would lie despite the assurance of "confidentiality."

Yet no red flags were raised in the mainstream press, which reported the study as gospel only a week before the March on Washington, with no follow-up questioning of any sort. It was left to the gay press to query the study's methods, especially the reach for geographical balance, when clearly it was the cities that had drawn gay men and women of the postwar generations. And the coincidence of the study's release on the eve of the high-water event of the gay and lesbian struggle was surely something short of innocent.

Winston and I had already been in Washington in late January, 1993, when I delivered the National Book Award speech at the Library of Congress. Then, only a week after the inauguration of the new administration, there was a quickness of spirit and an optimism that were palpable in the winter air, a sense that the nation had somehow survived the tyranny and arrogance of Reagan/Bush. Twelve years in the wilderness, and a legacy so bankrupt, so indifferent to human suffering, that one wondered if anyone could jigsaw the country back together.

The lifting of the ban on gay and lesbian personnel in the military had thrown us off-base a little. Most of our leaders in the community would never have called it the top priority. We all thought the President was going to announce an AIDS czar first thing. How could he not? We'd been waiting twelve years for some leadership in the epidemic—*any* leadership. What no one could have predicted was the tidal wave of homophobia unleashed by the military proposal: the pathological obtuseness of top brass, drunk on their misogynist prerogatives, coupled with the din of the Christian right.

One shrugged the usual shrug. Better that all their sewage and paranoia were aired in public, and not kept festering in churches and locker rooms and paramilitary boys' clubs. Decent people would surely see how crazy was the phobes' agenda. The head of the Texas Republican Party said that homosexuality should be a capital crime, punishable by death. And yet the country as a whole remained singularly ignorant when it came to fundamentalism. No one seemed to want to draw the circle that connected the World Trade Center bombing, the killing of a doctor at an abortion clinic in Florida, the standoff in Waco. No one in America was interested in the rise of worldwide fundamentalism, the politics of retreat from the modern world. Meanwhile, the Constitutional protection offered by freedom of religion had been used to obliterate the line between Church and State. The Christian supremacists wanted a Christian nation, thank you. Freedom of religion only if the free religion was *their* religion.

What was needed more than anything just then was leadership at the top: the President simply had to address the hatred. Using the bully pulpit, he could plead for tolerance and unity. Instead he held a news conference in which he seemed to suggest that gay and lesbian soldiers might be segregated, thus starting his own bonfire. He pushed the wrong button on civil rights. And though I didn't feel personally betrayed by the printed transcript of his remarks, the silence of the White House over the next several days was deafening. No clarifications, no bully pulpit. Little did the White House staff know that in our world silence had come to equal death.

I had been balking for several weeks about my own participation in the March, because there seemed a conscious wish among the organizers that AIDS be relegated to the background. It became increasingly clear that people with AIDS would not be on the rostrum—"because that's not what this March is about," as an organizer put it bluntly to a high-placed official with AIDS who wanted to speak. I couldn't get over

my own sense of disjunction. I kept envisioning a joyous parade of celebration, a giddy triumphal love-in where I did not
belong. I bore no animus toward the organizers for wanting
their March to be an arrival—no apologies for "lifestyle" anymore, but full participation in our rights as free citizens. I
would doubtless applaud that kind of March but didn't especially want to be there, relegated to the status of "a downer."

But the call went out with greater and greater urgency that
all of us had to *be* there, if for nothing else than to prove we
could rally the whole "one percent" of us to petition for equal
rights. Besides, the mood had changed since the hearings had
begun on the lifting of the military ban, under the chairman-
ship of Sister Nunn, a puffed-up Chicken Little who thought
the world would collapse if we let queers in. When we heard
that the President planned *not* to attend, not to address the
March at all, the simmering impatience made it plain that we
weren't gathering for a love-in for President Clinton.

Not to put too fine a point on it, one began to realize
that the question being raised—beyond equal rights, beyond a
cure—was, what did it mean to be gay and lesbian *now?* We
couldn't leave it to the scholars and the pollsters, that was for
damn sure. All those fights over the very name of the March,
which had flared up during the National Gay and Lesbian Task
Force conference in November. Bisexuals were clamoring for
inclusion. By the end of the conference it was being called
The March on Washington for Gay and Lesbian, Bisexual,
Transgender and Transsexual Rights, or some such agglomera-
tion. Perhaps one had to go to Washington simply to discover
if one still existed.

I weathered the flight pretty well. By mid-evening on
Wednesday we were in our rooms at the Park Hyatt, rooms
we'd booked in November. The message light was flashing as
we entered. My doctor had called from L.A. to say that the
results of the MRI on my brain seemed to indicate further

activity in the cerebellum. Unhappily the hospital appeared to have lost the x-rays from the previous scan six weeks ago, so there was nothing to compare the current pictures with. As if on cue, my head began to throb again. Tylenol barely made a dent.

We decided not to get up next morning for the dedication of the Holocaust Memorial, though that was why we'd come early. In January we'd toured the exhibit models prior to installation, and the staff had invited us to be present for the public unveiling. I was rattled by what I saw, even in miniature, and impressed by its defiant challenge of historical truth. The drumbeat of the Memorial was the constant question why: *Why was this allowed to happen?*

We gave our tickets to Jehan and Dwora, our lesbian friends from L.A. who were staying just down the hall. Dwora's mother had been in the camps and still bore the tattoo on her forearm. A couple of months before, in fact, she'd been hospitalized in Florida with heart problems. The doctor who examined her blanched when he saw the blurred numbers. "That's not what I think it is, is it?" he said, pointing at her arm. "No, I'm a fashion model," Dwora's mother replied with fine Viennese hauteur. "Didn't you know, this is the latest thing."

I woke up Thursday very slowly, glad we'd decided to skip the ceremony because it was cold and rainy out. Winston returned invigorated from an ACT UP action at the White House—three hundred people strong, a third of them women, demanding increased funding for AIDS. They had gathered in Lafayette Park, but the D.C. police wouldn't let them cross the street to the sidewalk in front of the Executive Mansion. As the cops grew more truculent and confrontive, Winston had shaken a finger at one of them. "You better behave," he warned, " 'cause there's going to be a million of us here this weekend!"

Already there was TV coverage of the ceremony at the Holocaust Memorial. Outdoors in the blustery chill, Elie Wiesel stood at the podium, hair so askew he appeared to have been tearing at it for days. Which he had been, actually, because another poll had been released that week, indicating that one in five Americans was ready to believe the Holocaust never happened. Wiesel had gone speechless in an accompanying interview, as if this knowledge was too much even for him, mocking as it did a half century of "witnessing."

But today he had reinvigorated his moral fire, gesticulating from the podium as he listed all the departments in Washington that *knew*. The decision not to bomb the rail lines to the camps in Poland, just miles from the military targets we did hit—all this he placed at Roosevelt's door. And he turned like an Old Testament prophet and pointed a quivering finger at the President. *Now what are you going to do about Bosnia?* he trumpeted, the connection clear to any child. He'd been there himself, seen all the madness and slaughter, seen it *again*. The question hung in the air that blasted him about like Lear on the heath. The President cast his eyes down, waiting his turn to speak.

A not bad speech, as it turned out, but fireless. One wondered what the world would be like if leaders had the passion of Elie Wiesel. Personally I'd rather have a leader tearing his hair out, than all the dulcet tones of a briefing with the National Security Council. Meanwhile there was little doubt, in my mind anyway, that the one in five who disbelieved the Holocaust was a real good Christian. Larry Kramer had remarked about the polls supporting the military ban, that no one would ever ask *Should Jews be allowed in the military?* But if such a poll were conducted, added Larry with laser precision, the Jews would probably lose.

We conferred with the doctor again by phone. In consultation with the infectious disease specialist, he was prescribing two more drugs for me to take along with the 566C80. We were to arrange with the pharmacist in L.A. to send them on to Washington by overnight mail. I was still feeling pretty rocky from Tuesday's chemo dose, and the throb in my head hadn't abated. But I had the wherewithal to tell him I'd proven allergic to one of those drugs last summer. He told me to go ahead anyway, starting with a quarter capsule, working up to dosage. The missing x-rays had finally been located, but it wasn't clear if they'd been looked at yet. Dr. Aronow, my neurologist, was on his way to Washington for the March.

Thursday afternoon we took a cab with Jehan and Dwora and made our way to the Jefferson Memorial. The wind chill off the Tidal Basin was daunting, so that we had to walk with our heads bent. Very few tourists had come this far today, but we waved to several queers we knew from Los Angeles. The city was filling up with us. Yet we had the domed interior practically to ourselves as we made our shivering circuit, reading Jefferson's words on the walls. The ringing condemnation of slavery, from a man who kept house slaves himself:

Commerce between master and slave is despotism. Nothing is more certainly written in the Book of Fate than that these people are to be free.

The groping toward the future, setting the course for Enlightenment:

. . . laws and institutions must go hand in hand with the progress of the human mind. As that becomes more developed, more enlightened, as new discoveries are made, new truths discovered and manners and opinions change, with the change of circumstances, institutions must advance also to keep pace with the times.

One wondered if gay and lesbian freedom was part of the change he foresaw—a man who probably hadn't the shred of a clue about the love that dare not speak its name. Did this faith in the constant betterment of the citizenry, the certainty that slavery would collapse of its own guilty weight, did its reach extend to peoples he couldn't conceive? His friend John Adams used to say that he studied politics and war so his son could study philosophy and his grandson poetry. Did Jefferson trust the poets to conceive a world he wouldn't even recognize, as long as it held to the first commandment, that *All men are created equal*?

What would the mood of the March be? Celebration or dissent—or both in concert? Would we leave no doubt that we were assembling here for patriotism's sake? Demanding that America honor its own vision of a place for everyone. No more invisibility. "I hold it," Jefferson wrote to Madison in 1787, "that a little rebellion, now and then, is a good thing, and as necessary in the political world as storms in the physical." Let us have a little rebellion then. Let the mood be so diverse that not even the most rabid phobes could say we were all the same—not godless deviants, nor a threat to their white-bread kids, but a people newly free, of every kind and stripe imaginable, with earrings to match.

We left the Jeff and had the taxi let us out at Dupont Circle, the heart of gay and lesbian D.C. Strolling up Connecticut Avenue, we could feel the gathering force-field of people arriving from everywhere. At Lambda Rising, the line to get into a *bookstore* stretched all the way to the corner. Storefront spaces had been leased up and down the avenue to sell buttons and tee-shirts and programs of the weekend's events. It was our first encounter with the tee-shirt that read STRAIGHT BUT NOT NARROW, proudly sported by a hetero couple holding hands and beaming at us, their brothers and sisters.

We ducked into a basement coffee shop to rest because

my leg was gimping up. The queer behind the counter promised us the best hot chocolate we'd ever had, a recipe specially made for the March. As we sat with our mugs at the counter, a gaunt man with a knapsack came in, dressed in combat fatigues and sporting a chestful of lift-the-ban buttons over his combat ribbons. He told us he had just driven in from San Diego with a carful of gay vets. He was weak and tired but ready to march. He and his group were camping out in a campground in Maryland, where they froze their nuts off the night before. He'd decided to bunk in a friend's apartment for the rest of the weekend, because "I don't want to go home sick."

That night we were meant to attend the National Minority AIDS Council dinner in the Great Hall at the Library of Congress. But by six o'clock I was being hammered by a migraine and a general air of malaise, like being seasick in calm waters, and the boat wasn't even moving. So we made our apologies and only heard later that night, in a flurry of telephone bulletins, that Larry Kramer and a group of ACT UPpers had disrupted the evening, preventing Donna Shalala from speaking. Our source, a member of the upper-echelon leadership, fretted and clucked that we mustn't be seen as disrupting free speech and assembly. I bit my tongue, glad that Larry was out there making noise. I was no fan of the Secretary of Health and Human Services, who had not so much as mentioned the A word since taking office three months before.

I finally connected with Larry by phone on Friday morning. No, he said, they hadn't prevented Madame Secretary from speaking. They'd simply passed around a bunch of leaflets, and then Larry and a woman of color had stood behind the Secretary at the podium, holding up signs that said DONNA DO-NOTHING. It was painful to think of the clash between the organizers of the dinner—some of whom I knew had fought long and hard to make this event happen—and the more

aggressive tactics of the street activists. It was billed as a Con-
gressional Dinner and titled "Our Place at the Table." But
there probably wasn't a more appropriate place to showcase
the tactical poles of the movement, our variety and our political diversity. And if push came to shove in the Great Hall,
there was no question which side I was on: "ACT UP, fight
back, fight AIDS!"

There was a documentary crew that had been following
Winston and me around for months. To us they seemed to
have shot enough footage to remake *Birth of a Nation*, but they
wanted a clip of us marching on Sunday. At this point I was
scheduled to ride up front on a trolley bus, provided through
the good graces of Marvin Liebman, the conservative movement's former darling and now *bête noire*. So the hobbled and
the ancient of days were to lead the throng onto the Mall.

Already, though, I was starting to question the wisdom of
my staying out all day Sunday, and to wonder if I'd come this
far in order to miss the parade. We told the documentarians
that they could accompany us to the Lincoln Memorial on
Friday afternoon, in case I had to disappoint them Sunday.
The Lincoln was a touchstone where we'd been planning to
pay our respects for months. The weather had grown mild
during the night, and with the last puffs of the passing storm
pillowing the bright blue sky, Washington had recovered its
gaudy airs of spring.

We piled all four into a cab driven by an Indian, who was
so friendly and eager to please that he could have been Aziz
in *A Passage to India,* oversolicitous but not without charm.
When we got to the Lincoln, I gave him twenty dollars and
told him to wait for us, ten minutes at most. My cabmates
gave me a look, as if I were throwing money away, at which
Aziz drew himself up with dignity and said, "You think I going to steal your twenty dollars? Don't worry, I be right here."

Monte and Lesli hoisted the equipment and followed me
and Winston up the steps. I'd been there before, but probably

not in twenty-five years. It had never struck me till now that Lincoln's memorial temple was the size and shape of the Parthenon; not by scientific measure probably, but feelingly at least, a most moving evocation of the daddy of public buildings, and thus of the democratic Age of Pericles that built it. And having made that connection, I further realized as I climbed the steps that the Jefferson echoed in its own way the sanctuary of Athena Pronaia at Delphi. There the most heartstopping ruin is the Tholos, a circular temple with only three columns still in place and a lintel above, but enough to reconstruct a classical heaven on earth—for us nineteenth-century types anyway. It seemed nicely fortuitous that the Parthenon and the Tholos both were temples to Pallas Athena, goddess of war but also wisdom.

There is nothing to match the Lincoln, in America anyway, for noble proportion and spiritual lift. You pass inside the Doric colonnade, and the columns in the entryway change to Ionic, with the ram's-horn capitals, a subtle shift to a more sophisticated style. Still, nothing quite prepares you for the power of the seated Lincoln—not the hundred cherry-blossom postcards that have passed through your hands over the years, nor even the patriotic swoop shots from helicopters that crop up in every civic documentary across the political spectrum.

You approach this massive marble pedestal, with the figure by Daniel Chester French looming above you. The toe of Lincoln's boot is off the pedestal, just above your head—a human touch that suggests a tall and rangy man who's too restless to sit in one place for long. And it's true, the eyes are haunted—staring out over the nation's city with a prophet's unshifting gaze, melancholy but also rock-solid sure that the nation's wounds would heal. No wonder it draws so many whose hope is faltering.

On the wall to the left is the Gettysburg Address; on the right the Second Inaugural. *With malice toward none, with charity for all.* I suddenly needed to stand on the spot where Marian Anderson sang her Easter concert, barred from Independence Hall by the D.A.R. I needed to honor Eleanor Roosevelt, who resigned from the organization and pestered Franklin to approve the Lincoln Memorial site. In the end Eleanor herself didn't attend, fearing to politicize the event even further. But there's a lovely detail in Joseph Lash's *Eleanor and Franklin*: Eleanor sitting quietly in the White House, the balcony doors thrown open, hearing the great contralto's voice as it floated over Washington.

All under the eyes of Lincoln, eighty years after the Emancipation Proclamation. Another quarter century later, and the tempered gaze of Lincoln—warrior and wise man—bore witness to the passion of Dr. King. I didn't think the Lincoln of my understanding would have had any trouble equating the Civil Rights struggle of people of color with the latter-day dreams of the gay and lesbian movement. There's too much compelling evidence in his own life—the bed he shared for four years with Joshua Speed above the general store in Springfield; the breakdown he suffered when family duties sent them apart—of the "dear love of comrades."[3]

In any case, I was choked with tears and in awe to be there, blubbering into my clip-on mike as the visit was recorded, a sort of super-video souvenir of a family trip to Washington. Standing in the shadow of the man who saved his country, it wasn't hard to see the religious right as a sort of Confederate belligerence. Only now they were hiding behind

---

3. Whitman's phrase. A most suggestive reading about Lincoln's relations with Joshua Speed is in Charley Shively's *Drum Beats* (Gay Sunshine Press, 1989). And note Shively's caveat: "The romantic cult of male friendship may have sometimes been completely non-sexual, but it provided a convenient form in which homosexual men could conceptualize their feelings for other men." (*Drum Beats,* page 88)

fundamentalist morality instead of States' Rights. And oh, how we needed a Lincoln to stand for equal justice and bind us all together again.

It was time to move on, because we'd promised Lesli and Monte a photo op in front of the White House. We trundled into the parking lot looking for Aziz, but he'd taken off with my twenty after all. I craned my neck to try and spot him, sure he was just circling the monument and would be back momentarily. Winston and Lesli and Monte rolled their eyes at my naivete, biting their tongues to keep from saying *I told you so.*

As we were coming up the street toward Pennsylvania Avenue, passing the Old Executive Office Building, we suddenly saw Larry Kramer, about to duck into a taxi directly in front of us. We raised a cry to stop him, and I clambered over to embrace him. Lesli and Monte, delirious at their luck, were already shooting. Larry introduced himself to Winston, and then we were off like a band of rebels, strolling past the Executive Mansion, Larry and I arm in arm. Though we talked by phone with a certain regularity, this was the first time I'd seen my friend in over two years.

We gossiped first, of course. The private Larry is a total *mensch,* warm and loving, the definition of decency. Those who were only familiar with his heroic public stance in the fight against AIDS, his Jeremiah role, often missed the heart's core of him. More than once during the weekend just beginning, I would hear his name taken in vain: *Larry goes too far. That's not the image we want to project.* And I'd reply what I always said: *What would things be like if we didn't have at least one like this?* More than a witness, more than a leader, in his own way like the Elie Wiesel who stood on the heath tearing his hair. With a constitutional inability to abide fools, was it any wonder that he shrieked and raged in this Swiftian Capitol of Fools?

It was a wonder to me that Larry could still fight like a

full-blooded warrior. Perhaps it was my own diminished capacity, fighting a pitched battle against the predations of the virus, that made me value Larry so. A stand-in for thousands of us teetering on the brink, someone who knew in his gut that a quarter of a million of us were going to die on Clinton's watch, even if the President proved to be a visionary leader in the epidemic.

Hearing us jabber and laugh, Winston was immediately reminded of Lincoln and Whitman. In the evening light the poet would be returning this way from the hospital, from his work as a wound-dresser. An aide would alert the President, and Lincoln would rush to the window to watch the passage of the country's premier bard. A poet who'd freed his own soul in the process of extolling the incalculable beauty of his country and its workers. No one has ever recorded an actual meeting of the two, though Whitman was as much in awe of Lincoln as the President was of the poet. But the well-thumbed copy of *Leaves of Grass* in the White House stood in moving counterpoint to the great funeral ode the poet would write on the death of his hero.

We stopped in front of the iron fence; beyond it was the great lawn sweeping up to the mansion. Larry pointed across Lafayette Park, where he used to stand as a boy in his father's office, watching the inaugurals. We became aware of a couple of corn-fed college kids, drawn by the documentary crew and unabashedly gaping at us. One of them got up the courage to approach Larry. "I think I recognize you," he said haltingly.

"Well, of course you do," I declared with a kind of avuncular pride. "This is Larry Kramer."

Larry squeezed my arm, adding, "And this is Paul Monette. You've struck gold."

The boys were from Lacrosse, Wisconsin—this was their first march, indeed their first trip to Washington. We asked them if they were the sum of the out queers of Lacrosse, and they shrugged their agreement. "There's another one," hazarded the taller of the boys. "But we're not sure if she made it."

It was the story of a thousand towns across the nation. Some of us making the trek to swell our ranks, ambassadors for the ones who could not come, who perhaps weren't out of the closet yet, even to themselves. Many among us coming out to family and friends by way of announcing they were on their way to the March, using this historic moment as a goad, as a diving board if you will. And so many others blowing their savings to get here, convinced that this watershed event would serve as a measure of their own freedom and self-regard, perhaps for the rest of their lives. Something to take home to Lacrosse, Wisconsin.

By the time we got back to the hotel I was reeling from exhaustion, the woodpecker still knocking at my head, my bum leg swollen to bursting. The overnight package had arrived from the pharmacy in L.A. I took out the three new medicines—Zithromax, Daraprim, Leucovorin, sounding like a trio of intergalactic villains out of *Star Trek*. I lined them up on the dresser across from the bed, staring at them. I was meant to start popping them right away, but I needed to somehow get used to them first. I was already taking thirty pills a day, not including the IV drip for CMV retinitis. How much medication could the body tolerate before the liver collapsed, or the kidneys? Not that I had any intention of rebelling, as I'd watched so many friends do—stopping all their medications cold, enough was enough, they'd rather be dead. And for a while at least they'd feel quite well, freed of the toxins and side effects of this sewer of drugs. And then they'd die.

I rested for two or three hours, husbanding my energy, readying myself for the evening ahead. A dinner party in Georgetown had been arranged to honor me, by straight friends who were tireless allies in the gay and lesbian cause.

Ties and jackets in place, Winston and Victor and I made our way to a flouncing Victorian row house off N Street. Our hosts, Bob Shrum and Marylouise Oates, greeted us with a fanfare of enthusiasm. The guest list was still in flux, but the Speaker of the House was definitely coming. Michael Kinsley would be right over as soon as he finished shooting *Crossfire*. And Tom Stoddard, head of the campaign to lift the military ban, would be a little later still because he was doing *Larry King Live*.

A rich mix of power politics, and to us outlanders a rare taste of being "off the record." It was implicit in the rough-and-tumble conversation over cocktails, this quick and brainy gathering of the savviest men and women, that the house off N Street was a journalistic safe house, no Mont Blancs and notebooks allowed. The talk was dizzyingly frank, about the filibuster and campaign reform and "how the President's doing." As a news junkie I could just keep up, and Winston murmured to Victor how refreshing it was that no one talked about movies. I thought of the Abolitionists, their heated meetings in parlors just like this one. (Lincoln, on being introduced to Harriet Beecher Stowe: "So you're the little woman who wrote the book that started this great war!") Or the Transcendental gatherings at Mr. Emerson's house in Concord. Philosophical politics.

At dinner I was seated across from Tom Foley, a witty and forthright man, appealingly modest and human, who came across altogether differently than he did on the Capitol steps, speaking *ex cathedra* into a thicket of network mikes. I couldn't bring myself to call him Tom, mostly because I preferred the rolling cadence of "Mr. Speaker." There was considerable conversation about the upcoming March and its potential effect on the hearings to lift the ban. (The consensus: no effect at all.) I shifted the ground of inquiry to AIDS, and the best and brightest of the journalists, on my left, reacted with genuine puzzlement.

"But you're going to get an AIDS czar eventually," he said, "and the funding's going to be there." The underlying question being, why were some of our people still protesting, and especially why so hard against the first President ever to be our sympathetic partisan? A very trenchant point; and how to explain what it meant that we'd been waiting not four months but twelve *years* and four months? We feared the epidemic, which had taken back-burner status after the military ban, would suffer from White House caution that the President not be perceived as giving "too much to the gays." (After all our railing that AIDS was not a gay disease but a global catastrophe.) Not that we doubted the President's personal commitment, but the polls apparently showed a nosedive whenever he reached out a hand to us. I withheld my personal trump card for hospitality's sake—that nothing could save me now, and yet I would still be out there railing for my brothers, unto my last breath.

There was talk among the straight folk at the table who worried that the March would hurt our cause. The argument went that Mid-America would be frightened off by our numbers and our rhetoric, and the inevitable press attention on the drag queens and the faeries. What they didn't seem to understand was that our March was for us first and not for anyone else's sake. Besides, we could scarcely have more enemies than we already had. And as one sequined man sporting a ball gown and a full beard opined to a minicam crew: "My wearing a dress doesn't infringe on anyone else's rights. And besides, it's after six. Time for evening clothes."

I found myself trying to explain to my end of the table my perceptions about the inadequacy of social-constructionist theory, which had reduced our ranks historically with sweeping abandon. And then this jerkwater poll that had pegged us at one percent. I told them about reading Sappho and the survival of feeling. They listened politely till one of the women, a superbrain in overdrive who'd managed the funding of the

'92 campaign in California, inquired with a nice candor: "Who's Sappho?"

I blinked like an aging professor long since put out to pasture. How could a sharp, well-educated woman not know the name of the supreme ancestor of *our* sort of women? I tried not to react like a stuffy prig, contemptuous of the spotty education of the young. I gave the poet her proper footnote, reciting some verses to back it up, then gave the floor back to political passions. I felt more nineteenth century than ever.

Back at the hotel I shook out a red capsule from the prescription bottle: Zithromax, ruler of the planet Toxo. I opened the capsule, dumped three quarters of the drug and swallowed the remnant. For the next twenty-four hours I'd be dashing in and out of the bathroom, lifting my shirt to examine my belly for rashy spots. I lay down exhausted, but not enough to sleep, reading my thriller till four A.M. One of the minor irritations of AIDS—*minor* as in not life-threatening, but even more *minor* on somebody else's skin—was an itching so intense that you wanted to flay yourself. No scratching seemed to quell it, though that didn't stop you tearing at it. Variously it had been diagnosed as eczema, as a side effect of one of my meds (but who could say which), and most comprehensively as "somehow connected with the virus." Meaning nobody had a clue. One of the doctors prescribed an unguent that seemed to help a little, only it left me feeling like a greased pig.

On Saturday morning I woke up shaky, realizing I hadn't been eating enough all week. 566C80, the drug that had held the toxo in check, had to be taken by mouth four times a day. But because it absorbed so badly, it needed to be taken with fats. So for months I'd been eating groggily in the dark—doughnuts and cheese and whole milk—helping along the five A.M. dose. I mostly ate ice cream for the waking doses, but that left my appetite stubbornly curbed. And even at that, the 566C80 wasn't doing the job anymore, so I had the feeling of losing ground with every doughnut.

I ordered a big room service breakfast, popped a full capsule of Zithromax, and encouraged Winston not to miss the
ACT UP action at the Capitol. For the first time really all
week, I started to feel trapped by AIDS. Mournfully I considered that this trip could be my last. I never doubted that I
needed to be here; but what about Italy and Jerusalem? The
world had shrunk quite suddenly in the last couple of weeks,
as I began to understand the intractability of the nexus of tumors in my leg, and grew terrified that my brain was clouding
up. I had yet to get through to my neurologist, though we'd
both left clusters of messages at one another's hotel. I sat down
to my melancholy coffee and croissants, feeling acutely left out.

I had a call from Richard Isay—the doctor who had re-
thought the psychoanalytic development of gay men, rescuing
us from stereotypes and defining our health in terms of self-
esteem. We had never met but had promised to be in touch
in Washington, hoping to find a free hour for a cup of tea. I
begged off by reason of general tottering and queasiness, and
Richard asked if there was anything he could do. I tumbled
out the tale of my leg and my brain, trying to be matter-of-
fact and not awash with self-pity. But that was exactly what
his ear was tuned to, and over the next two days he checked
in regularly. Not imposing himself but serving as an anchor,
especially in the absence of my medical team. A wound-dresser
indeed, like a Whitman of the psyche.

I read the *Washington Post* all the way through, checking
out the queer coverage. We were definitely the main news
this weekend, with coming-out profiles that let us speak for
ourselves about the witch hunts that characterized the military
ban. Meanwhile the Navy had released its appalling report on
the Tailhook scandal, all the woman-hating details, hoping that
it might get buried in the hoop-la surrounding the March.
These were the Navy geniuses who had tried to pin the U.S.S.
Iowa explosion on the broken heart of one gay sailor, only to
have to take it all back a year later. The same Navy that had

lied to Allen Schindler's mother, saying her son had been killed
in a fight, just an unfortunate accident. And one of his murder-
ers went free, and the other showed no remorse at his arraign-
ment. The truth would never have come out at all if Allen's
gay brothers in Japan hadn't blown the cover-up.

The same Navy that had turned whole villages in the Phil-
ippines into brothels, keeping all the girls clean for the delecta-
tion of the drunken slobs who came ashore. And this was the
Navy in which gay and lesbian people were not allowed to
serve because we might hurt morale.

I had a visit that afternoon from the writer Harlan Greene
and his lover, Olin. They had just been through a nightmare
battle over Olin's health insurance—a battle they'd won in the
end, but indicative of the Simon Legree tactics of the insurance
cabal that was always scheming to throw people with AIDS
out on their ear on the merest technicality. All of us lucky
enough to *be* insured lived in constant dread of a cancellation
letter. I'd had a case manager assigned to me some months
ago, and she kept me posted on how much slack I had. Just
the week before she'd left the information on my machine that
I'd used up $156,722 toward my million-dollar cap. I was safe
so far, but if the drug to save my eyes began to fail I'd have to
move on to a three-hour drip that cost twenty-six thousand a
month, just for the medication. Enough of those platinum
Band-Aids, and you could blow your cap in a year.

We were talking about Baptists, Harlan and Olin and I—
how the local parish tradition in the South had not always
been a breeding-ground for homophobia. It was very recent,
the assigning of diabolic status to queers. As usual, the hate-
mongering had paralleled the growth of our movement, a
pipe-bomb response to our coming out in droves. If only we
wouldn't talk about it, they said, they wouldn't have to mount
such a campaign against us. It was all our own fault. Meanwhile we'd just begun to hear rumors of the Nunn "compromise" that would come to be called "Don't ask. Don't tell."

Why couldn't we see they could live with us—Baptists and generals and pundits all—if we'd just stay in the closet? We can live with you if you'll just play dead.

Winston came back from "Hands Around the Capitol," ACT UP's exorcism of Congress. Fifteen or twenty thousand people had shown up, ringing the Capitol dome and grounds in a chain of protest, demanding increased funding for AIDS research and care. The event was a neat combination of witches' sabbath and shamanic levitation, culminating in a round of angry speeches by the likes of Michael Petrellis and Larry Kramer, whose coining of "Bill the Welsher" had thrown a new gauntlet down. "He's beginning to sound like Roosevelt and the Jews," said Larry. "Talks a good line and then does nothing." Bringing it round in a circle to Elie Wiesel, shouting his bitter *J'accuse* in the wind and rain. A circle of witness made tangible by the linking of all those hands.

On the Duty of Civil Disobedience, as the sage of Walden Pond called it. "Let your life be a counter-friction to stop the machine." And why? "I please myself with imagining a State at last which can afford to be just to all men. . . ."

When Olin and Harlan departed, I took to my bed again, beginning to feel positively neurasthenic. We'd been invited to several Eve-of-the-March receptions, including one which would preview the media spots for the lifting of the ban. A counter-friction, as it were, to the grotesque tissue of lies and hysteria which passed for the "family values" video making the rounds of Congress. But I couldn't pull it together, missing one gathering after another. Winston took care of me, soothing my imprisoned spirit. At nine o'clock I felt strong enough to get dressed, and we finally ventured out into the teeming throng of celebration, queers on every corner shivering with expectation of the day ahead.

I felt like their grandfather. Not unwelcome and not passed by, exactly—but bittersweet all the same, to find myself an elder before my time. Were it not for the virus I didn't doubt but that I would be capering in the streets myself. It was strange to be playing the reveler with Death so hot in pursuit, but somehow I rose to it. Probably because I was walking hand in hand with the man I loved. For here was the truly revolutionary act, to me the heart's core of what the enemy called the "militant homosexual agenda." Such a quiet gesture, really, no banners or slogans in evidence. Not proclaiming anything but a tenderness that had managed to endure the assaults of grief and sickness.

Jefferson made a great leap forward when he wrote the Declaration, amending the common-law notion of *life, liberty, and property* to the more felicitous *life, liberty, and the pursuit of happiness*. That was Winston and me. A careerist had asked us across a dinner table a couple of years before, "What are you working on now?" "Being happy," retorted Winston. A full-time job when you're living on a tightrope. Hard to choose a moment to represent all that, but perhaps that winter day, driving over the Continental Divide while I read him aloud the whole of Whitman's "I Sing the Body Electric." And finishing that, we suddenly saw on the blinding slope below the road a pair of wolves cavorting in the snow. We stopped to watch, silent a minute, till one of us remarked, "They mate for life, you know."

How to explain to a bigot so much resonance? The clasp of a hand on an evening's walk, the body electric, the mating of wolves. It's not written down in the militant agenda, and it isn't a "special right," as the current coinage had it when they passed the law against us in Colorado. It was simply what Jefferson promised, *pursuit of happiness*. As useless to pass a law against as to pass one against the wolves.

Later we joined a group of friends for dinner, straight and queer together around a table, trading stories about the weekend's exuberant parade. Toasting our health with a clink of ten glasses, but really toasting the fact that we were still here. Herb told us about the powerful appearance Allen Schindler's mother had made earlier that evening at the March on Washington Gala. With her plainspoken heart she thanked the gay and lesbian community for helping her to expose the Navy coverup. But more than that, she wanted to tell us all that people were wrong who thought we were weird. Such goodness and so much support in her grief had shown her what a loving tribe we were. "Thank you for my son," she said.

In the cab back to the hotel, Winston and I finally faced the obvious: I wouldn't be able to march tomorrow. Insistently I urged that he must go for both of us, with Victor and Jehan and Dwora; that I would be fine watching it all on C-Span, my leg propped up on pillows. He was just as insistent shaking his head no. He preferred to experience it all with me, however second-hand.

At midnight I finally connected by phone with my neurologist. Indeed he had seen the x-rays, and indeed there was new activity. Some swelling and edema of the lesion at the far edge of the cerebellum—a pain I felt about two inches behind my right ear—and indication of a new lesion, but this one just beginning, still very small. Had the 566C80 stopped working, I asked in trepidation, or had I developed resistance to it? No, it was just the absorption problem, nothing to panic over. I had a surreal vision of doubling my doughnut intake, liquefying whole boxes of Winchell's and feeding them through my IV line.

Dr. Aronow concurred with the rest of the team, that I should be adding the *Star Trek* trio to my regimen. As to allergic reaction, he thought the Hismanal I was taking to facilitate 566C80 would cover the new drugs as well. From the first he showed a fine capacity to calm my fears, and always with a jaunty assurance that he still had "other tricks up my sleeve." People with advanced toxo, he reminded me, were not giving lectures at the Library of Congress.

A reprieve then, though four weeks later I still make hourly forays to check my belly for allergy rash in the mirror above the sink. Part of the AIDS version of touching wood, a constant reminder that *now* is a temporary thing, all the more reason to seize it.

I got up at noon on Sunday, and Winston was already tuned to C-Span. The afternoon rally on the mall was just beginning, and we sat glued to it for six hours. The Woodstock energy was infectious and many of the speeches very moving, though we wished they'd pan the crowd more as it surged along the March route, past the White House and down Pennsylvania Avenue. It took seven hours to bring the whole sea of us onto the Mall, evening already before the last groups arrived. Later we heard a chorus of complaints from people who hadn't heard a single speech. That the marshals were unprepared for these kinds of numbers. That the ACT UP die-in—thousands of protesters falling to the pavement and playing dead for the seven minutes that passed between one actual death and the next, the plague's clock—had slowed everything down.

And the numbers themselves. A lesbian friend, veteran of the '87 march, was backstage when the Park Service arrived to make its estimate. They were notorious for undercounting, especially the likes of us. It was as if they'd learned their arithmetic from the pollsters who'd reduced us to one percent. My friend approached one of the youthful organizers and asked her where her negotiating team was. For this was the crucial bargaining moment with the Park Service, playing the poker of estimating crowds. A shrug from the organizers, who had no team in readiness. Giving the Park Service free rein to ballpark the lot of us at three hundred thousand, and this in the mid-afternoon as hundreds of thousands of us still flowed down Pennsylvania Avenue, nowhere near the Mall yet.

The D.C. police, no special friends of ours, put the figure at 1.2 million. The transit authority announced that four hundred fifty thousand extra riders had ridden the subway that day.

But the media picked up the Park Service figure alone as being the only "official" figure.

With so many people to speak at the rally, the participants were sternly limited to just a few minutes apiece, the entertainers to a single song. One of the early appearances was made by our friend Judith Light—who made the point that we were all here to teach our fellow citizens as well as every tarpit dinosaur in Congress. For years she'd been one of the movement's tireless allies, serving as the token straight on so many boards and dinner committees, emceeing so many events; she'd eaten enough hotel ballroom chicken to qualify her for combat pay. A big ovation before and after she spoke, Winston and I joining in all the whistling applause from our room-serviced exile.

Cybill Shepherd, the other ambassador from Hollywood, roused the crowd by recounting the story of calling her father to tell him she'd be here. "But wait—they'll think you're one of them," he declared with some concern. "Who cares?" she retorted breezily, to roars of approval all along the Mall. *Who cares?* became a battle cheer that day, perhaps because so many of us had had to confront the same anxiety from family and friends who fretted about our going public. *Who cares?* undercut the drama just the way Queer Nation did: *We're here, we're queer, get used to it.*

Urvashi Vaid, former head of the National Gay and Lesbian Task Force, gave a stirring rebuke to our enemies. Eyes flashing fire, she berated the "Christian Supremacists" whose own agenda was a determination to replace democracy with theocracy. She put them on notice in no uncertain terms that we'd be there to block them every step of the way.

Torie Osborne, who'd taken over the helm at NGLTF, was just as impassioned in her reaching out to embrace us as a united people. Halfway through she had a coughing jag, pounding the podium in frustration, gasping that she'd been working on this speech for four months. She didn't realize how human she sounded then, how much she embodied the halting declarations of so many of us, groping to find the words to set us free. Undaunted, fierce Amazon warrior that she is, Torie called for lemon, chomped on a wedge and finished to cheers.

Then she turned around and drew Larry Kramer to the podium. We heard later that she had done so under threat of arrest from the March organizers, still stubbornly asserting that AIDS wasn't what this March was for. But Larry gave his stump speech uninterrupted, a welcome gust of ferocity. Followed not long after by David Mixner, who spoke with a thrilling quaver about the outrage of the military ban, swearing a blood oath that there would be no going back.

There were too many lesbian comics, or too many not-ready-for-prime-time yet. Afterwards we would hear a lot of clucking about the woman who'd made an extended joke about doing it with Hillary. Didn't bother me, but then I was all for *nothing sacred* as a general rule for all such gatherings. When Congresswoman Nancy Pelosi stepped up to read Bill Clinton's letter of support—such small potatoes and scraps from the table—she was greeted by a din of catcalls from the crowd. Bravely she went on reading into the whirlwind, the words drowned out by a groundswell of withering disdain. Words by proxy were not enough.

It only made more telling the startling show of support we got from the NAACP. They told us they were with us and didn't duck the parallel with their own struggle. This was news, for they knew even better than we what an uphill fight they faced with the chorus of black preachers for whom homophobia was Gospel, who had spent a decade turning away from people of color with AIDS, to them the wages of sin. The writer Henry Louis Gates, Jr., would later make the telling point that Bayard Rustin, organizer and godfather to the '63 March on Washington, had demoted himself in the leadership ranks to avoid media scrutiny. All because he was gay. He stood off to the side, an invisible shadow, sacrificed to the greater good of freedom for his black people. Now at last the shame of one hero's silence could begin to be rectified by his *other* people, gays and lesbians.

If we didn't have Marian Anderson to trumpet us *Free at last,* we did have Michael Callen and Holly Near. Michael had been battling KS in his lungs for months now, and had actually been told by a medical professional that he'd be dead by March 1st. But somehow he'd made it to Washington, thin as a stick and on chemo himself. In a crystalline tenor he sang the song that had become a kind of anthem for a generation of lovers challenged by HIV. *Love is all we have for now,* goes the haunting refrain. *What we don't have is time.*

Holly Near—veteran activist, fighter for all women and the disappeared—gave forth with her own thrilling echo of "We Shall Overcome," harking back to the protest songs of the Weavers and Woody Guthrie. *We are a gentle loving people/ And we are singing, singing for our lives.* You could hear waves of people in the crowd joining the chorus, swaying with solidarity, survivors of the age of silence giving voice to their pride and dignity at last.

Perhaps my favorite of the speakers was Sir Ian McKellen, who offered a speech of Shakespeare's—from a play called *Sir Thomas More,* the collaborative effort of several playwrights that was never in the end performed. But Shakespeare's three pages, in which More confronts the mob of the King's men, constitute the only known example of the Bard's handwritten composition. In the play the King's men have passed a law forbidding "strangers" from settling in England—a slur against immigrants and a call for racial purity. Sir Ian stepped forward and trumpeted More's outrage. So they were going to forbid strangers, were they? And where would they go when the tables of history turned, when *they* would find themselves the strangers? It was an oratorical tour de force, giving historical

weight to the discrimination suffered by those who were
different.

All in all, a remarkable pageant of diversity. And from
where I sat, the flow of force was most tellingly toward the
young. Theirs was the first generation to grow up with the
promise of acceptance, at least from one another, and a measure of self-respect that constituted our hard-won legacy to
them. None of them had to be alone anymore, except by
closeted choice. As for passing the baton to a fleeter team, I
felt a measure of satisfaction—a family feeling, really—that
was scarcely quantifiable. But it wasn't one percent of me, and
was encoded in my genes for thousands of years, no matter if
it had no name. Or as Sappho put it, in love's terms:

> You may forget but

> Let me tell you
> this: someone in
> some future time
> will think of us.

For my own part, the invalid on the sofa, the phrase that
kept repeating itself as a kind of mantra was the title of Coleridge's poem, "This Lime-Tree Bower My Prison." The poet
had been waiting for months for a visit from his friend Charles
Lamb, beside himself with anticipation of showing Lamb the
glories of the Lake District. Alas, on the morning of his friend's
arrival, Coleridge "met with an accident, which disabled him
from walking during the whole time of their stay."[4] So he
mapped a route and sent the others out to experience the
earthly sublime. And all the while they're gone Coleridge sits

---

4. From Coleridge's prefatory note to the poem. See I. A. Richards, ed., *The
Portable Coleridge* (New York: Penguin, 1977), page 76.

in his garden-bower, which he ruefully compares to a prison cell, imagining his hiking friends as they follow his trail from mountain crag to sunset over the sea. Then the epiphany:

A delight
Comes sudden on my heart, and I am glad
As I myself were there!

Unexpectedly, the loving contemplation of his friend's adventure restores to him the beauty of his garden. The sublime is in every leaf, the dappled light on the walnut-tree: *No plot so narrow, be but Nature there.* Nothing so exalted in Room 404 of the Park Hyatt, but I felt the same heartened connection to the gathering of the tribe along the Mall—as if I myself were there. AIDS was my prison. Not very leafy, but sufficient to free the sympathetic imagination. Even in the throes of the viral assault, losing my body electric organ by organ, I could still make contact—no yielding yet to the isolation of dying.

And as the evening deepened and the rally stage was dismantled, I wondered how many had watched it all from the closet—that black garden where nothing grows, death-in-life. Would it spur them to a quicker recognition of who they were, watching us march a million strong? What would they muster of courage to free themselves? Torie Osborne had said that the real reverberations of this freedom march would be felt at the grass roots, when the million of us had returned home, there to confront the intolerance of neighbors and friends and family. Shaking the politics of Main Street.

Yet we all felt a certain reluctance to leave this crossroads moment of celebration, a recognition of the letdown that would inevitably follow in its wake. Myself, I would have to face my rage and sorrow that AIDS had been consigned to the back of the bus. The feel of second-class citizenship, even here at the top of the mountain. A fight that still had to be fought among us, over and over, so the sick would not be quarantined by a kind of AIDS apartheid. Noise would have to be made to ensure our full inclusion in the dream of a unified people.

But one thing was sure. Nobody left that marble city without a fuller grasp of what it meant to be gay and lesbian *now.* All the stereotypes lay in ruins. We didn't need our absent friend Bill Clinton to prove we had grown in political power. The torch had passed to the young, in the process lighting a million dark corners. The lonely frightened kids, trapped in fundamentalist families and all the lies of "Morning in America," would have at least a glimpse of what had gone on here, the counter-friction and the dear love of comrades.

In her peroration to the crowd, Urvashi Vaid had expressed it best in her charge to the heterosexual majority:

> I challenge and invite you to open your eyes and embrace us without fear. The gay rights movement is not a party. It is not a lifestyle. It is not a hairstyle. It is not a fad or a fringe or a sickness. It is not about sin or salvation. The gay rights movement is an integral part of the American promise of freedom.

Of course, what we would take away with us from Washington was also something much more personal. For me it began in a small town in Massachusetts forty years ago—a sickness of the soul about being different. And nothing more important, not breath itself, than the need to keep it secret. The stillborn journey of my life took off at last, the moment I opened the closet door. To know how dark a place you come from into the light of self-acceptance—it is to enact a sort of survivorship that leaves a trail for those who come after. But you carry that kid with you the rest of your life—wounded as he is by hate and lies—a shadow companion who needs you to free him.

And whatever is left of the hurt is washed away the longer you march, arm in arm with a comrade, rallying to the mus-

tering of the tribe. Until there's no dislocation anymore between the broken shadow of your past and the fully human
presence you've become. You have incorporated his pain and
come to understand that it is the very fuel that makes the torch
burn. No matter if they tell you you are only one percent, or
that two thousand years of your people have just been revised
and thrown to the winds. Nothing can dim the burning light.
You are home free, citizen and elder, one in a million. And
there is no America without you.

A ONE-WAY FARE

WE WERE ON one of those relentless cruises—a week from Monte Carlo to Venice, around the boot—where they dropped anchor once a day in a picture-book harbor and sent us off by tender to maul the local tourist goods. Warning us severely that the last tender would be leaving the dock at one-thirty—for the ship was sailing at two, with or without us. There was about all this a certain schoolmarmish insistence that we'd better stick together while ashore. For to be left behind would have the truants scrambling for a Cessna to drop us at the next port of call, untold demerits scored against us for violating the team spirit.

But as Miss Brodie was wont to tell her special girls, no one ever accused Anna Pavlova of having the team spirit. It was the *corps de ballet* that had the team spirit.

When we disembarked in Capri and wandered into town, Steve was content to commandeer a café table under the plane trees and drowse the morning away over coffee, adream in the vast cerulean of the view to the Bay of Naples. I had already had a run-in with the Ken doll who handled excursions. I'd told him I wanted to check out the ruins of Tiberius's villa, on the steep cliffs at the eastern tip of the island. He looked as if he'd much prefer to tell me where to score the best Majolica and cashmere, but coolly noted me on his clipboard and said he'd ask around.

About a half hour later he approached us under the plane trees. "Sorry, sir, we can't arrange it," he announced with a certain smugness. The emperor's villa was miles away, and the only way to reach it was by donkey on a dusty path. And all the donkeys were sick or in the fields or otherwise indisposed. As he went away pleased with himself at having foiled an insurrection among the sheep, I looked at my watch. Exactly two hours before the last tender.

"I think you better get going," declared Steve, looking up from a scribble of postcards.

"But what if I don't make it?" I retorted. "I don't know how far it is."

"Dr. Monette will make it," he assured me. Dr. Monette was his name for my literary self—or more generally, for the intellectual dabbling I was prone to, poring over maps and monographs of the classical world. To Steve, anything east of network television constituted scholarly work. Or as he would put it, wry and tender as he watched me at my desk, filling up legal pads with a novel in longhand: "Darling, nobody reads. Don't you know *that* yet?"

I zigzagged through the tourist hordes and started uphill through the lemony air of quarter-acre groves. Having no map was another sort of defiance, and anyway I soon reached a turnoff marked with a marble plaque, "Villa di Giove," with an arrow pointing up the donkey path that ran between the crumbling boundary walls of the lemon and olive growers. Too narrow for tourist buses, too rough and unpaved for mopeds. I struck a brisk pace and made my way in the noonday sun, not even any mad dogs or Englishmen for company.

After about half an hour I was still plodding east along the spine of the island, still no glimpse of the ruins on the heights. Spying a black-dressed woman feeding chickens in her back garden, I leaned over the wall and waved to get her attention. *"Scusi signora,"* I began, but hadn't got another word out before she pointed dourly up the steep path: *"Villa di Giove."* She seemed about as impressed by my destination as Ken the excursionist had been.

But I persevered, and in twenty minutes had left the hillside farms behind and entered the imperial precincts—wilder vegetation and here and there a tall umbrella pine to shade my way. I could make out now the stone remains of ramparts at the top, and I broke into a trot worthy of any donkey to cover the last half-kilometer. Arriving breathless at the first paved terrace, surrounded of a sudden by the bases of toppled columns, weed-choked cisterns, flights of stairs that stopped mid-air. The sun was blazing, but the quiet was incredible, a windless day where nothing moved except the lizards who scrabbled about.

There was no guide or guidebook available at the site, only a few tin signboards that gave a rough outline of the floor plan, all the labels in Italian. But frankly I didn't care by then, rapt as I was by the wrinkle of the azure sea below. "View" is hardly adequate to describe it. I felt as if the whole Mediterranean hovered in my ken, and the mainland shore across the water seemed a vision of the whole length of Italy.

I only knew a couple of things about this man who had lived here. That he had retired to Capri permanently in the latter years of his reign, leaving the running of the Empire to his underlings; and that he had hurled his enemies from this height, a thousand feet to the rocks below. A sybarite's dream of a place, then, unless you crossed the chief. I studied the ground plan and walked among the broken rooms, imagining them painted in the red and ochre of Pompeii. But the site had been pretty well denuded, sifted by archaeologists—no precious fragment like the Belvedere torso to be found; all of that hoarded long ago by the Vatican emperors.

And yet there was a fairly wide expanse of mosaic floor, forming a sort of triumphal path toward a grove of cypresses. Not the sort of mosaic fashioned into pictures; no coiled and rearing asps, no fighting lions or other imperial insignia. Just thousands of buff gray stones, each about a half inch square, and laid as tightly as ever after two thousand years. I crouched and ran a hand across its seamlessness, then followed the path to the cypresses which formed two stately rows on either side of the walk, leading perhaps a hundred feet to the sheerest edge of the cliff. No guardrail of any kind, just the vertiginous drop to the sea. Doubtless the place where the enemies were flung.

I cowered back from the edge, resting in the cypress shade as I tried to memorize the place. I assumed that the downhill trip would be quicker, but I'd already passed the first hour and more. The time squeeze throbbed in my belly, affording me no leisure to spend a lazy afternoon at this lookout, picnicking in the cypress shade. All I had was a couple of speeded-up minutes to commit this glimpse to memory. I turned reluctantly away, looking back over my shoulder as the vision receded, framed by the cypress alley.

Then my downcast eyes took note of the breaks in the pavement where cypress roots had burrowed beneath the mosaic, fissuring the surface till the beaten path was littered with rubble like a scatter of dice. I knelt and picked up a loose square of mosaic, noting how its structure was in fact a rectangular wedge, whose half-inch square of exposed surface concealed the depth of the stone, a full inch of foundation below. Presumably this shape made it easier to pack them tightly together to make a solid floor.

I didn't even have to think twice, swiftly pocketing the stone and casting about for another to bring back to Steve. The first law of ruins—*Never take anything away*—surely didn't apply to me and my thumbnail souvenirs. The winter rains would only wash away these patches of broken mosaic, burying them in the mud and weeds. No team of archaeologists was going to bother reconstructing a footpath. And yet I felt oddly guilty as I made my way over the terraces and started downhill, prickling with the worry that what I'd done was just a matter of degree. A latter-day Lord Elgin, who "liberated" the Parthenon friezes and sailed them home to England, just to keep them safe. Or those whole temples carted off stone by stone by the Germans, for the purposes of study. Leaving the ancient sites as bare as the plains of Troy.

Ruins get ruined, there seems no way around it. Even Rose Macaulay—in her sinfully delicious book, *Pleasure of Ruins*—announces with a certain breezy shrug that every ruin is in constant flux:

> . . . one cannot keep pace: they disintegrate, they go to earth, they are tidied up, excavated, cleared of vegetation, built over, restored . . .[1]

But that only makes more urgent one's imagining, projecting the self along the "ghostly streets" of what she calls "the stupendous past." She doesn't say how long one ought to stay and contemplate, to make the place one's own. But fifteen minutes hardly seemed enough, especially as I stumbled down the rock-strewn trail like a mad donkey, racing the clock to the harbor.

Of course Steve was right. I made it with moments to spare, looking dazedly off the stern of the tender as Capri floated away. And even then it felt like a dream, my time in

---

1. Rose Macaulay, *Pleasure of Ruins* (New York: Thames and Hudson, 1984), page iii.

the emperor's ruins. I have in the four years since managed to preserve the memory intact, or almost. The cliff-edge eagle's perch, the sweep of the sea below. What I have left besides that blinding abruptness is this fragment of gray stone rubble on my desk, a single piece of the jigsaw.

And of course the story of my adventure—so vivid in recollection that it convinces after all that fifteen minutes on the heights sufficed to make it mine. And yet, so perverse is the drift of memory, that at a certain point in time I had a change of emperors, giving credit for the Villa di Giove to Hadrian rather than Tiberius. That may seem like a minor glitch, though a century separates their two reigns. But it gave me leave to populate the pleasure-palace on Capri with Hadrian the aesthete, builder of libraries and founder of the Atheneum, the gathering-place for the intellects of his age. And to remember his passion for Antinoüs, the joyous comrade of his heart, who drowned in the Nile in his twentieth year. Temples went up in his memory, and a hundred sculpted portraits besides, to assuage an emperor's grief.

So it made a kind of cockeyed sense, to picture Hadrian retiring to his widow's peak on Capri, in melancholy contemplation of stolen love. It certainly fit my fantasies, with Steve about to follow Roger through the portal from which there was no return. Imagine my confusion, then, when I sat down to write this story and turned to my classical reference books. No mention of Capri in any of the entries on Hadrian. I grew so anxious, so unable to tell the tale without proof, that Winston brought me home from the library a book-length bio of Hadrian. Capri was not in the index, or anywhere else. A skim of the text kept throwing up details—that relations between the emperor and the boy went on for nine years (and remember, the boy was drowned at twenty); that in fact there were more than five hundred busts and statues of Antinoüs still extant, more than we have of Hadrian himself. Pictures of

Hadrian's villa at Tivoli. The Pantheon. The obelisk on the
Pincio.[2]

I was mistaken, that was for damned sure. And in the process had learned more than I wanted to know about the times,
preferring to see them through the mists. I'd always understood that Hadrian had had a peaceful reign, no foreign wars
or barbarous invasions. But it seems he proposed to found a
pagan colony on the site of Jerusalem, compounding the mess
by outlawing circumcision. The ensuing revolt was fearfully
bloody, leaving the Jews bereft of a homeland.[3] And still I had
no answer to who had built *my* villa on the cliffs. I began
leaving messages, slightly crazy, for various scholars I knew;
and was starting to dial Garry Wills in Illinois, sweating like a
graduate student, when the name popped into my head: Tiberius.

Of course. 14–37 A.D., a hundred years before Hadrian.
A misanthrope, Tiberius, whose "reign was one of terror, with
spying, prosecutions, vengeance and suicides. His life has been
painted in the darkest colors by Tacitus . . ."[4] Well, at least it
began to make sense, those enemies flung from the eagle's
perch. I'd always had a difficult time trying to jibe such ruthless abandon with my image of Hadrian, the aesthete queer.
And I suddenly felt absolved of any lingering guilt about stealing two chips of paving stone from the Villa di Giove. A bad
guy's lair.

But it's certainly made me reconsider what's real in the
facts department of my travels. They are seamless to me after
all, tight as a Roman mosaic, those moments of thundering
clarity on various peaks and temple sites. In the end they have
come to be strung on the single thread of my sensibility, a sort

2. Stewart Perone, *Hadrian,* New York: W. W. Norton, 1960. Frankly I hate to
proffer the footnote, given the rank homophobia that permeates the discussion.
3. Howatson, *Oxford Companion to Classical Literature,* page 258.
4. *Ibid.,* page 498.

of pearl necklace of wonders—and not very many of which allowed me much more than the fifteen minutes I copped on Capri.

Oh, there are places I've gone back to numerous times, and always with a fervor to recapture, to drive the experience deeper—but that is something else entirely. And there have been occasions when I've found myself in the neighborhood of one of those places barely glimpsed, and so took a second shot. Santorini for one, the lip of the volcano; or the cloister of Saint Trophime in Arles. Second visits that were usually more in the nature of happy accidents than the keeping of a blood promise. We may make any number of silent vows to return, to relive the flash of the sublime and maybe even the glint of a lost self. But it's like Frost's oath at the fork in the wood, swearing he'll keep the road not taken for another day—

> Yet knowing how way leads on to way,
> I doubted if I should ever come back.

We are booked for a one-way passage, no return.

The older we get, the more does it all sink in. That the trail of grain we've dropped in our wake like Hansel and Gretel has been snatched and eaten by crows. A postcard arrives from one of these magic places—dashed off by a friend who may even have gone there at our insistence—and the frozen picture is suddenly more real than our own recollection. Surely the tower was on the other side, and couldn't you see the ocean from the top?

All the more reason to get your fifteen minutes right, so the place will remain indelible, no matter if the fog of memory mirror-reverses the tower. We're told that Gertrude Stein always sat with her back to the view, so everyone else would have to face her. She also says somewhere that all views pale after fifteen minutes. She may be right: that we can't take in too much sublimity at once, or that our nature is to reduce all experience to banalities, shrink the world to postcard size. Myself, I'm after a different sort of quarter hour—a willed intensity that meets its destination halfway, at a certain romantic pitch. Not the historian's way, by any means. Or the archaeologist's, who tries so hard not to clutter the site with preconceptions; dispassion before all else. And certainly not Gertrude's way, whose life was a sort of monumental site all by itself.

But then if it takes a whole lifetime for you to get to Mont-Saint-Michel, you have already watched the tide come rocketing in at thirty miles an hour—in your head, anyway— a hundred times. The towering rock in the bay has been waiting for you as long as you have been waiting for it. The spiral climb through the medieval quarter, the looming church at the summit, a labyrinth of stairs to reach it. What's to disappoint? The wild romantic burnish you've endowed it with turns out to be the truth. In a minute you have peopled it with a flock of white-robed monks, and you seem to float in air as lightly as the Archangel himself when you gaze up at his gilded figure high at the top of the roof, seeming to spin on tiptoe, the pirouette of faith.

Who needs dispassion?

Not that it always works, by any means. In Noel Coward's *Private Lives,* when Elyot and Amanda come face to face on their separate balconies, they're on their honeymoons with different people. They talk inanely about what they've been doing since their messy divorce. Elyot stutters through the tale of his trip round the world, Amanda nervously filling in the gaps.

> AMANDA: And India, the burning Ghars, or Ghats, or
>   whatever they are, and the Taj Mahal? How was
>   the Taj Mahal?
> ELYOT: Unbelievable, a sort of dream.

AMANDA: That was the moonlight, I expect; you
 must have seen it in the moonlight.
ELYOT: Yes, moonlight is cruelly deceptive.
AMANDA: And it didn't look like a biscuit box, did
 it? I've always felt that it might.
ELYOT: Darling, darling, I love you so.[5]

There's always that chance that you've traveled across ten
meridians, only to find a biscuit box. It happened to me once
in Greece, where otherwise all holy places met my expectant
heart with garlands of laurel. Steve and I lay stupefied with jet
lag in an Athens hotel, waiting to board the rusty tub that
would take us round the Aegean. Dr. Monette decided there
was time to rent a car and drive to Sounion, the cape round
which all ships made their way to Athens, the headland
crowned by a temple to Poseidon. We ended up in a belching
Austin mini that smelled like a farmer's truck, as if the previous
lessee had been a flock of chickens.

The suburbs of Athens went on and on, concrete-slabbed
apartment blocks that looked like barracks. By the time we
reached the sea we were at last in open country, though it was
scarred by the grisly villas of the rich. I began to have that
anxious gnaw that we wouldn't be back in time, the bane of
so many of my expeditions.

Then we came round a bend, and there it was on the crest
of a hill—a small hill, as it turned out—its eleven Doric columns honey-colored in the heat shimmer of the summer sun.
We parked and walked up past a shady *taverna* to the brow of
the hill, and instantly I had to rein the poetry in. Not that I
was expecting another Parthenon; and the eleven columns are
no less eloquent for being built to human scale. But I'd always

---

5. Noel Coward, *Three Plays* (New York: Grove Press, 1979), page 209.

assumed it perched on a high cliff, rather like the Villa di Giove, so its beacon fires would be visible halfway to Crete.

No such height. Really, a bare stone's throw from the water below. And the columns themselves were covered nearly top to bottom with the names and initials of previous visits, scoring into the soft stone. Not exactly tagged by the spraycan sort of graffiti, but violated all the same. Unguarded, unprotected, an easy drive for a day-tripper. *Not enough, not enough,* my heart cried out.

But I withheld from Steve the hollow of my disappointment, especially since he'd had enough after *five* minutes, and moved to take cover in the arbor of the *taverna,* nursing a Greek beer. I wouldn't let him order any food—for Christ's sake, he wanted a salad, an invitation to crypto and who knew what other microbes. It was why we traveled by ship in the first place: to exercise some control over the food, as much as to accommodate a steamer trunk of medicine. I sat with my back to the temple, surely a blasphemy against the sea god. Glancing over my shoulder, it wasn't so bad; at least you couldn't see the hieroglyphs of graffiti at this distance.

And so we wended our way back to Athens in a smut of traffic. The pang of Sounion had mostly receded within a day's sail, as we crossed the Sea of Marmara to Istanbul. But a jumble of myth still rattled around in my head for a couple of days, the ashy taste of failure. For it was at Sounion that Theseus was meant to change his ship's flag from black to white, to signal his father the king that he'd made it home alive from Crete and the Minotaur's cave. When he forgot to change the flags, grief-stricken Aegeus threw himself off the Acropolis, to be dashed on the rocks below. Of course all of this transpired in mythic time, pre-history, and who knew if I had the facts right anyway, mostly a rehash of Mary Renault. But the feeling persisted, like a low-grade fever, that I'd somehow flunked my exam in ancient history.

The curative for which is prescribed most movingly in Cavafy's cautionary poem, "Ithaka"—

> As you set out for Ithaka,
> hope your road is a long one . . .
>
> May there be many summer mornings when,
> with what pleasure, what joy,
> you enter harbors you're seeing for the first time;
> may you stop at Phoenician trading stations
> to buy fine things,
> mother of pearl and coral, amber and ebony . . .
>
> Keep Ithaka always in your mind.
> Arriving there is what you're destined for.
> But don't hurry the journey at all.
> Better if it lasts for years,
> so you're old by the time you reach the island,
> wealthy with all you've gained on the way,
> not expecting Ithaka to make you rich.
>
> Ithaka gave you the marvelous journey.
> Without her you wouldn't have set out.
> She has nothing left to give you now.[6]

It is hardly Sounion's fault, in other words, that it doesn't quite measure up to one's lush specifications. Perhaps the disappointments have their purpose too, to balance all those blurred mirages with a laser dose of focus. And anyway, it's not the end of the journey yet. So you reset your sights and keep going.

---

6. C. P. Cavafy, *Collected Poems,* translated by Edmund Keeley and Philip Sherrard (Princeton Univ. Press, 1975), pages 35–36.

I needn't have fretted at all, really. The next day out of Istanbul, we turned south along the coast of Asia Minor, passing the windswept site of Troy, now utterly vanished. We stopped in the channel that lay between Lesbos and the mainland, then headed inland through miles of tobacco fields to the citadel of Pergamon. I didn't know a thing about it—neither a smatter of fractured history nor the slightest image, mirage or otherwise—and so I quickly reverted to the studious schoolboy, clamoring over the ruins and checking out every cistern, every cornerstone. It was just as Cavafy foretold, the pleasure and joy of an unknown harbor.

So we circled the watery cradle of the Aegean, dolphins leaping about our bows, and nothing looked remotely like a biscuit box. The voyage even provided one of those rare second sightings, at Delos, where Roger and I had idled away an afternoon six years before. An island that's uninhabited, the birthplace of Apollo, and a major center of commerce in the ancient world because it served as a crossroads for ships bound east or west. We landed just after sunup—Steve and I, his mother and sister—on the very first tender launched from the ship. So there was a moment when the first group of us had it all to ourselves, an unbelievable stillness as the sun caught fire and dazzled us with a whole world of ruins.

Just inland from the harbor there's the wreck of a colossal statue to Apollo. Two boulder chunks, one still faintly tracing the shoulders and chest of the god, the other his hips and buttocks. And if you needed another reminder that *nothing gold can stay* (Frost's rueful formulation), the guidebook reproduces a drawing from 1673. Apollo still had his head then, and the pelvis supported his thighs, almost to the knee. Too big for the plunderers to carry away, and left to the surer plunder of wind and rain. *Memento mori* for days.

But the lake of the god's birth remains, weed-choked now, more mud than water. Guarded by lions sent in tribute from Naxos, a row of heroic marble beasts sitting on their haunches, mouths agape with roaring. Disintegrating in front of your eyes, two of them legless and propped up on steel rods, and yet the guardian stance and the roaring somehow seem immutable. Though the sun god has long since departed—streaking the sky in his chariot, shedding gold in his wake—the watch of the lions remains at full attention, profound as the saints on Gothic cathedrals awaiting the Second Coming.

But enough slides of my summer vacation. You get the picture: a boy who never went further afield than a two-weeks' cottage at Hampton Beach, just across the border in New Hampshire. All the while reading too many books about faraway places with strange-sounding names. And I know exactly why I've been pulling out the scrapbooks these last weeks, because the journey has suddenly stalled. The road doesn't go any further, the bridges are all washed out, or maybe I've just gone overboard in a squall. So I gather all my memories of the places barely glimpsed, the stamps that litter my passport, and wonder if all together they prove that I went the distance.

I understand that there isn't a final exam for this. The map studded with pins is purely subjective, and in any case nowhere near the driven pace of travelers like Paul Theroux and Bruce Chatwin, who seem to live exclusively on trains and tramp steamers, or riding camelback up the sacred mountain. And needless to say, they don't stop for fifteen minutes once they get there; they stay until they've drunk it to the lees. Graham Greene in Haiti, or making the rounds of the leprosaria in the Congo. D. H. Lawrence in Italy, Joan Didion in El Salvador. Exploring the places where people live beyond the end of the road.

Of course it's no secret why my ticket has expired. Because of AIDS, the borders have narrowed further and further, till whole continents are now in the red zone. Forget Africa, or China or India, the Middle East, any place equatorial. Even when I was asymptomatic, still juggling a hundred T-cells, I crossed off half the world for being too dirty. Couldn't eat the meat or the milk or the fruit, let alone drink the water. There was something almost xenophobic in all this, an overcaution that looked at the world through a glass bubble of paranoia.

As if one couldn't get just as deadly sick in one's own backyard. A doctor friend has warned me never to order water in a restaurant, or anything with ice, comparing such recklessness to dipping a cup of water from the Nile. For a year and a half I haven't touched a shred of lettuce. As soon as I heard the only safe way was to put the leaves in a sinkful of water with a tablespoon of bleach, I went off salads entirely. Odd, because I always thought of myself as rather intrepid.

Not anymore. What amazes me now about the memory of Capri is that stride up the rocky path, especially the final burst to the summit. That's the real Dr. Monette, prepped for so many years by his daily trot on a treadmill, never out of breath for a minute, no matter how steep the trail. Now it's all come down to this swollen leg of mine, too much exertion reducing me to a hobble by day's end. Even with the addition of a stretch surgical stocking, refined last week with a garter belt that girdles my waist and clamps the stocking in place. Till I am something of a cross between an atherosclerotic old lady and a genderfuck chorus boy in a kickline. Winston calls the orthopedic shop—staffed as it is by a trio of sturdy Eastern European women—Frederick's of Poland.

We still hope the new chemo is going to work, shrinking the KS lesions in the lymph system so that the dammed blood will circulate again, flushing the swamp of edema. And I mustn't complain too much, because I've made it to the next breakthrough—a chemo regimen that has no debilitating side effects. After four doses it has flattened out and faded most of my surface lesions to mere gray smudges, but it hasn't yet drained the swamp. That tenacious "leg thing" again, so far eluding all the tricks of oncology, leaving a whole division of us limping about.

This may be the best we can do with it, sighs Dr. Thommes, pressing his thumb to the swell above the knee, leaving a dent in the flesh. *Just keep it from getting worse.*

These strange plateaus of dying, where you bargain away your dancing days as long as it doesn't get worse. If that sounds like rank self-pity, it's not intentional. I've watched this swelling go up and down for nearly a year with a certain abstractedness, testing my body mechanics, still trying to outwit the creep of complications. Staying in charge, riding my illness as if I was breaking a horse, till lately anyway. If there's one specific moment when I *got* it, all my denial suddenly in tatters, it would be last month in the Canadian Rockies.

Still on course for Ithaka, even then. A new direction—due north—and a territory unexplored, at least by the likes of me. We flew to Calgary and then headed by car for Lake Louise. We put up at the old railroad hotel at the southern end of the lake, a drop-dead view from our room of mountain peaks on either side and the glacier itself pouring slowly over the northern ridge. It was the runoff that had created the opalescent green of the water in the valley. Picture-perfect.

And for some reason I had neglected to factor in my limitations. Though I could stroll along the shore for a quarter mile or so, hiking was out of the question. But that was the way I'd always done it before—trailing up out of the valley in hiking boots, bound for the high country. In Yosemite with Roger, straight to the top of Bridal Veil by switchback. Or the Lake District, the high green hills above Grasmere, no one else at the top. The hiking having the salutary effect of letting the mind go blank; or if lost in thought, with none of the petty clutter of the quotidian.

So what was I supposed to do now, give all that up for a lawn chair and a lap robe? Waiting for a nice cup of bouillon,

to be served by one of these ridiculous waiters in Swiss costume. The big event of the day being the blowing of a ten-
foot Alpine horn on the near shore, "God Save the Queen"
barely distinguishable from "Amazing Grace."

O Canada. Winston and I both did our damnedest not to
let it separate us, trying to keep me from feeling left behind.
He who had the force and energy to climb these peaks to the
sky, but mostly chose to stay by me. We pretended it didn't
much matter, the view from the top. And made the return trip
by way of Banff National Park, the road through the vast old-
growth forest quickened by elk and bighorn sheep grazing the
verges without fear. We were a zoo to them, I suppose. There
certainly wasn't any doubt who was caged and who was free.

Home again after six days' northern passage, we finished
the Canada roll of film on the front porch, mugging in our
tuxedos because we were on our way to a benefit. It was those
prints that couldn't lie, that seemed to show the first faint trace
of the skull beneath my skin, no matter how wide I grinned.
Not that I wasn't grateful for the journey, energized even, but
this was the trip that would always bear an asterisk, proof that
I couldn't leave AIDS behind. I remember the exact evening
in '84 when César announced, *I've traveled enough*—a man
whose life map was a veritable pincushion of countries tra-
versed and holy sites. Whose only destination out-of-town
from there on in—besides Death, that is—would be our
house, a quick shuttle hop from San Francisco. I remember
promising Roger we would get to Paris again somehow, even
after he'd lost his sight and mostly lay curled asleep, Puck
on the floor beside him as if they were having a sleeping
contest.

Did I believe that promise? I suppose I didn't. More than
anything it served as a goad to memory and happier days. Besides, I saved my deepest passion of disbelief for the opposite
scenario, that our traveling days together were over—that we

had no way anymore *to change our ideas,* as the French would put it. Grounded.

I was beginning to dread that I'd have to venture alone along the next leg of the journey, but not prepared to concede the point. For the lie to my intrepidness was this above all: that it wasn't any fun to be anywhere without someone to share it. Hardly the sort of attitude that will see you solo through the jungle or up past fourteen thousand feet. I'd certainly done my share of that sort of thing in my closeted days, sitting hugging my knees as I took in the view from the High Corniche, or the coral chambers visible far out to sea from a hilltop in the Bahamas—lonely, lonely, lonely. No escape and no vacation.

Somehow it all got intertwined with being in love. It surely was no coincidence that traveling changed from the dutiful checklist of masterpieces, confided to my journal to somehow make it last; changed the day I met Roger, like everything else. After that it didn't signify anymore what the destination was. Paris through his eyes, England through mine, and then we were in uncharted waters, sailing along in our sub-sub-compact—the deal being that the one not driving was navigator and guide. Maps so cumbersome they needed a charthouse to be laid flat, flapping about till neither of us could see the road ahead. Or reading aloud the deathless prose of the Green Guide so we'd know what to look for when we arrived.

Once, on a delirious ride through fields of lavender and the dusty green of olive groves, I read to Roger from Ford Madox Ford, his love song to Provence:

> It is no doubt that illusion [of the permanence of London] that made my first sight of Provence the most memorable sensation of my life and that makes my every renewal of contact with those hills where grows

the first olive tree of the South almost as memorable.
It is as if one wakened from a dream of immortality to
the realization of what is earthly permanence.[7]

Or the sudden detour into Wales to check out the ruins
of Tintern Abbey. I bought us a pocket Wordsworth before
we left Bath, and Roger in his mild voice recited the great
poem of return:

LINES

COMPOSED A FEW MILES ABOVE TINTERN ABBEY,

ON REVISITING THE BANKS OF THE WYE DURING

A TOUR, JULY 13, 1798

We crossed the mouth of the Severn just after Bristol—its
tall industrial chimneys clouding a sulfurous sky—and entered
Wales. Immediately the landscape changed, electric green and
pastoral, as if we had crossed the border into a reverie.

When we reached the Abbey itself, there were no other
cars and no guard in the kiosk. I hadn't realized how lofty the
ruins would be. Though all the stained glass had been ripped
from its windows when the abbeys were routed, the tall
Gothic windows were filled instead with the green of the hills
surrounding. The roof and its beams were gone, long burned
away, a conflagration that took the wood paneling off the
walls, along with the choir stalls and the altar. But the bare
stone of the great nave was otherwise unbroken, buffered by
graceful side aisles. And someone had had the aesthetic sense
to mow the grass that had overrun the floor paving, so that
you walked through the soaring ruins on a carpet of velvet
lawn.

---

7. Ford Madox Ford, *Provence* (New York: The Ecco Press, 1979), page 88. A
reissue of Ford's text, first published in 1935.

It was such a perfect realization of the poet's faith, the Divine-in-nature—a pagan temple now, given over to the earth, monument to the ecstatic urge of life:

> . . . something far more deeply interfused,
> Whose dwelling is the light of setting suns,
> And the round ocean and the living air,
> And the blue sky, and in the mind of man . . .[8]

Roger and I wandered around with our heads tilted skyward, tracing the noble arches and gables against the cloudless blue. I must've stopped at a windowsill to jot a note in my journal—still trying to freeze these spots of time, maybe even outdo the poet himself. Such vaunting self-assurance in those days. I finished mid-sentence, hitting the wall of clichés perhaps, but mostly trying to catch up with Rog. Behind the church proper were the briefer remains of the dormitories and kitchens and stables, easier for the anti-papist vigilantes to pull down and obliterate. You could just make out traces of a cloister, with a well in the center.

I don't remember what sparked it, but suddenly I was in a panic that I'd lost Roger. I called his name in the green stillness, then started racing about—the camera like a millstone round my neck, my journal as dead as Latin. In seconds I had him tumbling down a well, or crushed by a falling gargoyle. No other tourists, still no guards, and the fear of being alone more overwhelming even than the worry. I kept crying out, through a choke of sobs, the green river valley and the godless church as alien as the moon. *Please, please, don't let him be hurt.*

And then he emerged calm as you . please from the restrooms by the kiosk, his smile fading as he walked toward

---

8. William Wordsworth, *Selected Poems and Prefaces*, ed. Jack Stillinger (Boston: Houghton Mifflin, 1965), page 110.

me, seeing the wrench of relief in my tear-streaked face. Of course I felt a fool by then, but he gently soothed my residual hysterics, promising over and over that he was fine. I still don't know where it came from, some long-forgotten memory of being separated from my parents in a crowd. But eight years after Tintern Abbey—when Roger was running the gauntlet of tests at UCLA, on the brink of his diagnosis—the rattle of the same terror overtook me like an old wound leaking pus. Except this time it went on and on, unrelieved, for the whole twenty months of his illness. And I often think that Tintern Abbey was by way of an AIDS rehearsal, a premonition of mortality that I had no words for yet.

The incident doesn't appear in the postcards we sent, nor anywhere in the travelogue we regaled our friends with. Tintern Abbey still stood in its emerald vale—stands there yet—consecrated to Pan and a host of nymphs and satyrs. The "something far more deeply interfused" lies in its green reassurance that nature stands apart from the sully of human fret and bother. In other words, the canker in the rose was all mine, baggage I brought with me. What I would lose if Roger disappeared was the reason to go in the first place.

This is a problem inherent in mixing up the journey with being in love, but it's the price you pay for being a certain breed of romantic. The "earthly permanence" slaps you in the face, mocking your little span of seasons, your fleeting embraces.

So it ought to come as no surprise that the world is vastly bigger than all your travels, but it does. Maybe it's like reading. Starting as far back as my twenties, when my nose was always in a book, I recall the particular shiver of melancholy, realizing I wasn't going to get through the whole of Henry James. Or Dickens or Proust or Tolstoy. There just wasn't time. Even at a clip of a hundred pages a day, a vivid sense of my own limits. But I shrugged it off, assuming that was one of the boons of getting old. A rocking chair on a white picket veranda, dozing your way through *The Wings of the Dove.*

And then to be startled to find that life has become more interesting than books. Besides, you get by perfectly fine on the ones you *did* read. Even as the details start to go, you can talk with practically anyone on sheer enthusiasm alone, from *Persuasion* to *David Copperfield.* In the end it becomes enough to say how marvelous something is, how true and close to the bone. After all, the people you're talking with have mostly put off from the shore of books themselves, paddling through the shoals of life with barely a thriller on the nightstand.

Is that how traveling goes, once you realize you're not going to make it to Benares (those burning ghats) and Machu Picchu? Do you just fall back on where you've been, embroidering your stories till everyone you know has heard them twice over? Or do you prove you've gone the distance by becoming a small authority on the 7th Arondissement, or all the bronzes of Florence? Making up in sophistication for what you lack in mileage. Well, whatever works to dull the longing for what you've missed.

And anyway, you've eavesdropped enough in cafés to hear a lifetime of witless remarks by people who scarcely notice where they've been, just a string of hotels and bad meals and the shopping terribly disappointing. Like the man who approached the moral philosopher Sidney Smith[9] and rapped his walking stick on the pavement. "You see this stick, sir?" the gentleman boasted. "This stick has been around the world."

"Indeed," replied Smith. "And yet, still only a stick."

Sometimes what catches your fancy is the oddest detail, yet it leaves a deep notch on your walking stick. In Crete in '84, Roger and I took a solitary tour of the wrecked Minoan

---

9. 1771–1845, founder of *The Edinburgh Review.*

palaces from the Bronze Age. Four altogether, I think, and all destroyed at once, circa 1400 B.C. The palace of Knossos being the most impressive, excavated and partially restored by Arthur Evans—throne room intact and the dolphin frescoes swimming in a stairwell. So many rooms and corridors that one story has it that Knossos itself was the Labyrinth of myth. And all obliterated, so the theory went, when the great volcano blew in Santorini ninety miles away, causing a tidal wave that reached Crete within six minutes, wiping out the whole Minoan civilization. Stupendous past indeed.

Contemporary scholars have questioned the drama in all of this, convinced that the decline of the palace culture was slower, a matter of centuries. True though that may prove to be, I find I prefer the *feeling* truth of tidal wave and wipeout. But then, don't come to me for the facts.

Some miles inland is the palace of Phaestos, high above the Mesara Plain, and exquisitely unrestored. We had that one all to ourselves as well—pure luck of the draw in the Ithaka business. Up the great stone staircase into a maze, most of it leveled to the bare foundations. And in the rubble of a store-room, according to the pidgin English of the guidebook, had been found the so-called Phaestos Disk. The sole surviving evidence that the Minoans had a written tongue as far back as the Second Millennium B.C. (but still no clue what it said).

Later that day in the Heraklion Museum, our eyes glazed over by rooms full of potsherds, we came to the dusty case where the Phaestos Disk, the thing itself, was on display. About the diameter of a Frisbee, the clay perhaps two inches thick, and the whole surface deeply incised with pictographic signs laid out in concentric circles. There were learned guesses as to what it might say, but none held water. No one knew whether it was meant to be read from the center outward like ripples, or spiraling in from the rim.

All I know is that it possessed me, holding me fixed as Roger moved on to the snake-goddess fetishes. For a little while there I actually convinced myself I could crack it. Without the slightest training in hieroglyphics, this layman who could scarcely keep Hadrian and Tiberius straight thought he could best the experts. Spellbound, getting nowhere, I must've stood there fifteen minutes waiting for a brainstorm. And then I left it with that same look over my shoulder, regret/desire, with which I'd walked away from the brink in Capri. Knowing how way led on to way; knowing I'd never be back.

The feeling returned full force a couple of years later, when a friend who'd studied Greek at Oxford told me about his tutor. An ancient dusty man with patches, wreathed in pipe smoke, whiskers in his ears, and fluent in an astonishing range of dead tongues. He happened to mention one day that he was working harder than he ever had, trying to translate all that was left of some nameless forgotten language, a slew of clay tablets somewhere between Sumerian and Aramaic. For decades he'd tried to pass it on, but it was too hard for even the best of his students. Apparently you had to know everything else to get that far.

The truly lost, the undeciphered, constitute a kind of backlash as you gather in the world, destination by destination. I never expected in my lifetime to watch a country disappear—and then the bloodshed exploded in Yugoslavia. But wait. What about our day in Dubrovnik—Steve and I—the pristine medieval port, pride of the Adriatic? Clocktower and lion fountain, steep cobbled alleys radiating off the square, old women watering their windowboxes, or leaning on the sills and smiling like cats dozing in the sun.

Do the places you've visited still exist in your head if they're reduced to smithereens? Are they anything more than postcards after all, doomed to go to the grave with you? People sigh over Beirut, the Paris of the Middle East, a distant look of confusion in their eyes, bereft of words. Or the old Tibet of the monks, the vision of Lhasa riding the clouds, the palpable Zen of desirelessness. Before China began the genocide.

Now we hear that the Muslim fundamentalists in Egypt want to rid the place of all Dynastic monuments, from the Pyramids and Sphinx to Karnak and Abu Simbel. Graven images and, sin of sin, built before Mohammed. Or the leveling of the temples in Cambodia, of *everything* in Cambodia, a whole country committing suicide till the ground was sown with salt. There is no end to this, of course. The world is coming apart at the seams, and traveling at all becomes more rarefied every year, increasingly a fixed route to places certified intact and free of terrorists.

Elitist almost by definition, a sort of Orient Express in spirit if not in fact—brass-fitted and bottled snowmelt and turndown service at night. The planet as theme park, Disneyized. McDonald's at the intersection of Boulevards St. Germain and St. Michel, across from the ruins of the Cluny Abbey, itself built on the ruins of a Roman bath.

My cousin Harry came back from Orlando in a cosmopolitan rapture: "First night we had dinner in France, next night in It'ly, then England . . ."

And his wife piped up, "Don't forget Japan."

This is not the same, itinerary-wise, as Marlene Dietrich standing on the rail platform, face like alabaster in the night, declaring: "It took more than one man to change my name to Shanghai Lily."

The sure sign of a travel snob: *been there, done that.* The world-weary affectation, preferably in profile and white dinner jacket. It's not till much later, the end of the line, that you realize what a wandering quest it's been, willed or not.

And when life brings the journey to a halt—by incapacitation, or the fares grown too stiff, or maybe just sheer exhaustion—it doesn't matter whether you're my cousin Harry or Shanghai Lily. No extra points for mileage covered or trekking the inaccessible. The bags go up in the attic, you let your passport lapse. You can actually feel the loss of motion. Then you look out the window and realize here's your Ithaka: home at last. Cavafy again, the final stanza:

> And if you find her poor, Ithaka won't have
>   fooled you.
> Wise as you will have become, so full of experience,
> you'll have understood by then what these
>   Ithakas mean.[10]

Not that I've come to a full stop, not quite yet. Two weeks after Canada we were on our way up the coast to Big Sur, the place I've returned to most, the one that never disappoints. Not fifteen minutes but days and days over the course of two decades, till I could trace every mountain slope and rocky point blindfolded. But if Canada broke the denial that AIDS could be left behind, the Big Sur trip took it further— a conscious flight from the war zone, hobbling like mad, bandages trailing like streamers. An old friend had died of AIDS the week before—and then a week after, one of my doctors. Both were diagnosed at the same time I was. We'd been on the very same tightrope without a net, like the Flying Wallendas, and now I was teetering all alone. I went to Big Sur to convalesce a failing spirit, but knowing full well it would be no cure.

Still, the first two days were a breath of air. By dint of prosthetics—Polish stocking and garter belt—I managed the full two miles to Molera Beach, where I sat propped on a driftwood log with Winston at the mouth of the Big Sur River. Neither of us haunted by goodbyes or the last look over the shoulder. The wildness didn't mock us or embrace us. It simply let us be. But by the third day there was business

---

10. Cavafy, *Poems,* page 36.

that wouldn't wait—matters of the will, the charitable trust, the selling of the house in a mummified market. Death and Taxes. Necessary though it may have been, it left us shaken and out of sorts, squashed by details. We hiked back to Molera the next day, more somber, more distant. The landscape withholding entry into the full sublime—the hawk's slow circle, the pound of the sea, the place where the deer lay down their bones.

This last a sanctuary that Robinson Jeffers stumbled on while hiking one day, a dappled glade with a clear stream running through, the ground littered with rotting bones and antlers—where the old and wounded came to die.

> I wish my bones were with theirs . . .
> . . . why should I wait ten years yet, having lived
>   sixty-seven, ten years more or less,
> Before I crawl out on a ledge of rock and die,
>   snapping, like a wolf
> Who has lost his mate?—I am bound by my own
>   thirty-year-old decision: who drinks the wine
> Should take the dregs; even in the bitter lees and
>   sediment
> New discovery may lie. The deer in that beautiful
>   place lay down their bones: I must wear mine.[11]

It's more than a bleak refusal to kill himself. It's that trapped detachment that goes with being human and dying alone. As if I were looking at Molera Beach, the place that has always stopped my heart, from behind a wall of glass. As if I were looking at the memory of it and not the thing itself, all the while wearing my bones like a straitjacket.

---

11. Robinson Jeffers, *Selected Poems* (New York: Vintage Books, 1965), pages 100–101.

Next day we recovered our equilibrium at Tor House in Carmel, the house that Jeffers built with his own hands, boulder by boulder from the shore below. A site I hadn't visited in ten years, and then with Roger. So: one of those rare second chances. A shipshape house like a captain's quarters, with the bed by the window that Jeffers had chosen to die in from the beginning. (Otherwise used as the guest room, its true purpose withheld from the guests for politeness.) Out in the garden, the housedog's grave: *Haig, an English bulldog.*

But more impressive than anything else, the tower at the foot of the garden—Una's tower, built for his wife as a private retreat. A tower out of a Viking saga, or from the Irish cliffs of Moher. Not thirty feet high but grander than any watchtower, and built forever, its sea-smooth boulders more massive than even the house stone. With a secret stair inside, besides the main one spiraling up the outer wall to Una's dayroom. A unicorn's lair, with a narrow double window looking out over the bay—where Jeffers swore he saw a merman once, in the turbulent winter tide, breaching the white-capped swell for a moment's look at man's estate, then diving down again.

And the final climb to the parapet, with only a swaying chain for a railing, a hawk's perch where the wind blows through you. Mythic in a word, but a myth whose gods were profoundly mortal, a man and a woman in love. No mixup here: Winston and I had found our way to a monument that was in feeling equal to the twining of our two hearts. A place of inexpressible human permanence. You come away with the understanding that Jeffers's work is twofold—the poems and the tower—like the source of two rivers.

Then coming back to L.A., and still so restless. Some part of me long since finished voyaging, yet compelled by a near atavistic urge to be a moving target, to make Death have to run and catch me. The crisis of it came upon me unawares, unbidden. Winston had made plans, months before, to attend the annual gathering in the wild of a group of radical faeries.

Nine days at the start of August, and the only time in the year when we were apart. I had no right to ask him to forgo it, in part because I wasn't sick in bed, but more because it was something he'd still have when I was gone.

This isn't to say I wasn't terrified to be left to my own devices—a late relapse of the Tintern Abbey panic and its progeny, the helpless waiting for Roger and Steve to die. Except in my case now the waiting was for me. There was nothing for it but to stay in motion.

So I asked Victor, who'd fled to Europe with me after Steve died (sniffling our way through cathedrals), and again last summer to Big Sur when Winston was off in the woods. Left it to Victor, my last best friend, to check out the availability of Alaska, a cruise along the so-called "Route of the Glaciers." Only to find that every ship was booked to the gills. For Alaska was suddenly terribly in, the prudent alternative to IRA bombs in London, tour buses strafed in Cairo, the hijacked Mediterranean.

We had to settle for a waiting list, then a cabin the size of solitary confinement in the bowels of the *M/S Sagafjord*. But you won't be spending time in your room, the travel mavens assured me. *Oh yes I will,* I thought, *nearly all of it in fact*. My role model being Simone Signoret in *Ship of Fools,* overripe with her own mortality, who didn't quite speak anyone else's language, returning home to certain imprisonment. No question about it, I needed the cabin more than the ship.

Then at the last moment there was a cancellation on the Officers' Deck at the top of the ship: somebody must've punched his ticket early, keeling over into his Samsonite even as he packed his woolens. We left for Vancouver on the 28th of July, Winston having packed me for every eventuality, practically sewing my name in my socks. With a vast pharmacopoeia of medicine in tow, an igloo just for the IV bags, steeled for a grilling at the border. Mr. Monette, could you tell us why you're traveling with forty syringes?

But Victor and I squeaked through without a hitch, and in any case I had a letter from my doctor listing all my meds though omitting to mention AIDS. This medical report had been required by Cunard regulations, to be turned over to the ship's doctor on embarkation. We were still surveying our cabin, with its own private terrace above the lifeboats, bags not yet delivered, when the doctor himself appeared. A Swede who seemed to sport a permanent curl of distaste beneath his weedy mustache, who pointedly avoided shaking my hand. He'd clearly been clued in about the "A" word, and was most concerned that our ship's insurance would cover evacuation by chopper.

"These little ports we visit," he said amiably, "they've never heard of these drugs you're taking. They're not equipped for . . ." Words failed him, but not that curl of distaste.

So he left us to our lepers' quarters. Never having caught *Ship of Fools,* apparently, or he would have had Oskar Werner for *his* role model. With his steely blue eyes and stiff-spine air of melancholy, who ended up in a shipboard liaison with the Countess (Signoret) because they shared a sense of last chances, the common tongue of irreversible fate. I did not expect our Doctor Strindberg to be slipping into our cabin for a little mid-ocean action.

But at all events, that is how it happens that I am still on the road to Ithaka, having long since learned what Ithakas mean. A landscape more staggering every day: hundreds of miles of forest right to the water's edge, lighthouses blinking time, range on range of snowy crags. And the glaciers themselves—forbidding, unyielding, cracking like rifle fire, calving icebergs into the floe-strewn bays. Not to take anything away from such exaltedness, but the main characteristic of Alaska—at least to us in Cabin 141—is the blankness. Rather like that blankness of a day's hike, nothing else in your head, nature over mind—desirelessness, with or without the Zen.

Thus we abjure all shore excursions, lacking the team spirit, and in eight days have managed to meet not one of our fellow passengers. I have seen one eagle perched in a treetop, and the barest wave of a humpback's tail as it dove back under. No mermen of course, but these are not times that lend themselves to heroic sightings. I feel no abiding curiosity about the people or their history, having had my fill of Manifest Destiny and the tribes that have perished beneath its wheels. At least I won't get the facts wrong. No, the blankness will do just fine.

The rest is the force of memory, with its tricks and elisions, but all my own till my lights start winking out. My various fifteen-minute epiphanies have been in the nature of chance encounters, revealing things I didn't know I was searching for. Strung together, they provide a kind of window into what endures, even as it melts or shakes to bits in a quake or falls to Huns and marauders. That is how *I* see it anyway, the trail of a single traveler. Certainly no one is going to follow my peculiar progress as if it's a useful guidebook from A to B, let alone Z. My fact-free cultural map is harmless enough, no threat to the vast theoretics of ethnographers and linguists, art scholars, all those patient diggers.

My own map is freely drawn in sand, and the tide is coming in. I am unencumbered of any grand thesis, mostly ignorant of antithesis, but achieving a private synthesis all the same, though I can't really put it in words. No tablets left behind to be deciphered. Only this: the cost of a one-way fare is life.

Not that my random journey is going to help me die any easier, except insofar as I don't feel cheated, not of the world out there anyway. My hoard of destinations suffices to let me imagine the rest. Srinagar, Cuzco, Persepolis: name it and something flickers, like and not like somewhere in your head, a paradox yes, but devoutly wished.

And I will not give up a scrap of it without a fight. For years I used to save postcards, dozens of them from everywhere, because they did a better job of freezing time than my poor blind-spotted camera. Eventually they filled the secretary in my bedroom, a jumble of disorder, potsherds from a myriad of civilizations. Last year I started to use them for notecards, filling three or four at a time and tucking them into envelopes, my only real correspondence anymore.

I don't usually choose my views with any forethought: someone will get the Piero frescoes in Arezzo or a silversword cactus from Haleakala, House of the Sun. I linger a little before parting with anything Greek, however, directing these more pointedly to friends who might get a flicker of their own. I understand I am spending my loose change, scattering it to the four winds, but careful not to lighten my ballast so much that I will float away.

No, I am only sending out announcements of my last stand. When I will be taken kicking and screaming from this phenomenal world, intractable to the last, ferocious in surrender:

> With all my might
>   My door shall be barred.
> I shall put up a fight,
>   I shall take it hard.
>
> With his hand on my mouth
>   He shall drag me forth,
> Shrieking to the south
>   And clutching at the north.[12]

Big talk, but what do I know? I may go yet like Jeffers in the bed by the window,

---

12. Edna St. Vincent Millay, *Collected Poems* (New York: Harper and Row, 1956), pages 206–207. Lines from "Moriturus."

When the patient daemon behind the screen
of searock and sky
Thumps with his staff, and calls thrice:
"Come, Jeffers." [13]

About three months ago the consummate traveler, Freya
Stark, died at the age of one hundred. "The first Western to
journey through many regions of the Middle East," [14] volumi-
nous writer and scholar and wit. Spoke Turkish and Arabic
before she hit puberty. Sometimes rode for weeks by camel
and donkey. Fierce anti-fascist, and hardly a country she didn't
write about.

In her ninety-third year, a reporter asked her about that
final port of call. She was busily on her way to Spain, but
stopped to give it some thought, for Death was doubtless the
ultimate foreign country. "I feel about it," she said at last, "as
about the first ball, or the first meet of hounds, anxious as to
whether one will get it right, and timid and inexperienced—
all the feelings of youth." [15]

Exactly. When no amount of intrepidness will see you
through, nor the globe in your study that fairly bristles with
pins. You are suddenly in the clutch of a new adolescence,
watching your helpless body change before your eyes, hating
every blemish, waiting with dread to see where you will next
put your foot in it. The no-way trip. Be glad, I suppose, if
your morphine dreams at the end are a slide show of your
voyages, superimposed on the shining faces of all your beloved
companions who've matched their steps with yours. No telling, since that final Northwest Passage is all one-way. Postcards
not available; or else they get lost in the mail.

---

13. Robinson Jeffers, *Poems*, page 54.
14. "Dame Freya Stark, Travel Writer, Is Dead at 100," *New York Times*, 11
May 1993.
15. *Ibid.*

Meanwhile, incredibly, there are miles to cover yet. Just now we are cruising the Kenai Fjords, a starfall of scattered islands worthy of *The Odyssey,* the lairs of giants and the call of Circe, the flashing sun on the water leaving us muzzy as the Lotos-Eaters. Tomorrow we land in Anchorage. Long past journey's end, however you look at it. But the road isn't done till it's done, and so you go on till Death catches up. Soon enough. But you wouldn't have missed these islands, surely, even if they're the last. Oh, especially if they're the last.

GETTING COVERED

I

THERE'S THIS TO BE SAID for being marginalized as an artist, laboring in obscurity, year after unsung year—you get to develop a voice of your own, unfiltered by fawning overpraise or the exigencies of the marketplace. It doesn't mean you don't want it all: your name in lights on Forty-fifth and Broadway, a window display at Rizzoli, a GAP full-page in tee-shirt and baggy pants. But when it doesn't happen and doesn't happen, you begin to see you've got nothing to lose. This is a good place to start taking more and more risks with your work, assuming you don't fall into bitterness and envy of the overpraised, thus chewing your own spleen like a raven. And even then you might write something true, bile being as good as ink. But mostly you will have avoided being smothered by what Gore Vidal calls "bookchat."

When I was a kid we used to have a conundrum in the schoolyard, an early warning of the Hobson's choices life would set in your path. *Would you rather eat one bowl of Eisenhower's snots,* we would ask the unsuspecting, *or two bowls with*

as much sugar on top as you like? There was no right answer of
course, but our schoolmates, ever prudent, would usually opt
for the second choice. Thus in later years would they find
themselves ready for bookchat.

During the years when I was writing poems exclusively,
there was no bookchat for miles in any direction. Budding
poets would fob themselves off on one another with reams of
Xerox copies. If recognition was to be courted at all—nothing
so vulgar as fame—it was by way of being elevated to the
Pantheon, with Frost and Auden and Lowell and the Misses
Moore and Bishop. Otherwise one masticated the crumbs as
best one could. Especially a penciled scribble at the bottom of
a *New Yorker* rejection slip: *nice work* or, even better, *send more.*
One dared not hope that the unsigned bit of reassurance had
come from Howard Moss himself, the poetry wizard of that
particular Oz.

Still less did one dare to dream of an actual *acceptance:* a
poem in the magazine, interleaved between the pages of an
Isaac Singer story, with a Booth cartoon on the facing page.
One could only imagine reaching that height of cosmopolitan
splendor.

It was very rare to see a poet interviewed in print, except
in the littlest magazines of the trade. No poet ever sat for a
radio call-in or, heaven forbid, a television appearance. If you
were *really* well connected in the poetry biz—a poetician as it
were—you could aspire someday to the *Paris Review,* the series
called *Writers at Work.* But that was about as far as one could
go, publicity-wise. One's ambition and competition were on
a higher plain entirely: tilting at the windmill of anthologies,
holding out for a place among the centuries, rubbing shoulders
with Keats and Emily Dickinson.

Poets weren't part of the gossip at large. Remember, this
was a time when dinosaurs still roamed the earth, before the
invention of *People.* Yet even without a central clearing-house

for personal trivia, poets knew all the gossip about one another, almost by osmosis. The status of various rocky marriages; who was on lithium, who was not; how drunk they were for their reading at the Y. A viper's tongue was part of your poetical equipment.

At twenty-eight I executed a U-turn and made for the ranks of the novelists. Only to be marginalized ever more pointedly, because I published a novel populated almost exclusively by gay men. It didn't feel like such a revolutionary move, and I was supremely unaware of being part of a vaster historic thrust to create a literature on the margin. Of course my novel was largely ignored by those poisoned malarial waters that constituted the *mainstream*. But I did fall into the babbling brook of the gay alternative press, whose own gathering presence announced the arrival on the scene of a wave of gay and lesbian writers and artists. *Out* writers and artists, which distinguished us from our forebears and all their brave euphemisms to keep from being labeled *queer*. With all proper deference to Whitman and Proust and Genet and James Baldwin. Perhaps it's more accurate to say that we were the first generation post-Stonewall to be out and proud in our work, no apologies. But who knew that we were a whole new literary movement?

The alternative press practiced a kind of anything-goes journalism, vital and irreverent. There was the *Gay Community News* in Boston, the *Blade* in Washington, the *Bay Area Reporter* in San Francisco. These and several more were at the urban core of our presence in cities across the country; and *The Advocate* still in its youth but fighting to be a truly national voice.

Cub reporters would call, and you could hear them typing furiously to get it all down, or covering the receiver to bellow for silence in some noisy downtown loft. Gay news was a palpable thing, its presses running on overtime. The questions they asked were political and frivolous by turns, but in any case the opposite of the turgid academics of the *Saturday Review of Literature* and its ilk. Because my central character was a thinly disguised portrait of Dietrich, the interviewer could give it a nice camp spin, asking me to theorize as to what made an icon gay. They wanted to know my sun sign, and whether I'd ever been to Fire Island. Who was my boyfriend, and did I believe in monogamy? And my favorite color? Green, with purple a very close second.

Yet underneath it all there was a far more serious matter to be pondered: *Was there a gay sensibility?* The question would be asked in a variety of guises—but always uncertainly, as if fearful that an affirmative answer would leave us all ghetto-ized. Yet I agreed there was, without any hesitation, even if I had to stumble to put it into words. Yes, we wrote with an outsider's angle, and we wrote from a place of invisibility. More than most people—especially the straight white male variety—we had to invent ourselves out of whole cloth. There was a certain naivete about us, pugnacious but with a wild aim, that marked the delayed adolescence which attended our coming out. One thing was sure, this gay sensibility was a good deal more complicated than doing fabulous windows at Bendel's or sewing bugle beads for pop divas.

We asked more questions than we answered in those early years of the seventies, as a literature slowly began to coalesce around our fundamental uniqueness as a tribe. Gay Christianity, gay teen suicide, gay substance abuse, gay Meccas, and gay families. Our differentness had as many departments as *Time* and *Newsweek* put together. It was only in 1973, after all, that we ceased to be a disease, when they finally dropped us from the diagnostic manual of crazies. We were still a fair decade or more from the tangles of Political Correctness and the locked horns of Queer Theory, the essentialists butting heads with the social constructionists. So there was a window of time where we had the freedom to self-define, a sense of ourselves as recording and witnessing what had only been shadows before; present at the creation of something unheard of.

This situation gave us the ground to consider whether gay men and lesbians could ever be brothers and sisters. Did the passions of radical feminism dictate that we would always be on separate tracks? As to the further business of whether a truce between gay and straight could ever be achieved, the jury was still out on that. I can't begin to say how many times I was asked: *Are you a gay writer or a writer who happens to be gay?* Definitely the former, though many of my friends weren't ready to bite that bullet yet. To them, *gay writer* sounded more political than literary.

Sometimes the reviews and interviews exhibited a certain bitchiness, or a pettiness nursed by free-lance journalists who had a novel or two of their own in a desk drawer, longing to be clothbound. Sometimes, to the contrary, the critical judgments of the gay press were far too lenient, so much puffery. There was a tug-of-war between a genuine critical rigor and a well-meaning enthusiasm that owed a good deal to the shiny domain of the press agent.

But at least the coverage was by our own, and so we gave it a lot of latitude. I sold first serial rights to *The Gold Diggers* to *Blueboy* magazine, which printed the chapter about Sam the hustler in two parts, two consecutive issues. It was a bit of a stretch, I admit, to see my pages of limpid prose tucked between photo spreads of donkey dicks and fantasies of getting it on with telephone repairmen. The aspiration to Isaac Singer and the Booth cartoon still had its hooks in me somewhere. But then, there was a certain camp rightness to the *Blueboy* juxtaposition—definitely a turn-on for a man like Sam, and no less so for his creator.

Memory has mercifully blurred the details, but I still cringe when I think of the interview I gave to *After Dark,* a sort of all-purpose entertainment guide from the seventies with lots of pictures of dancers stripped to their tights. Gay was the unspoken subtext, though it dared not speak its name. My interviewer was the redoubtable Norma McLain Stoop, an eccentric gargoyle of a lady whose gushing fealty to show biz was nonetheless infectious. So excitable she could barely sit in her chair, maybe fifty-five behind all that rouge, and with a proprietary feeling about her boys in the business. What the cruel and limiting argot of the times would have called a *fag hag*, which did no justice to her overflowing loyalty and sense of fun.

We talked for a whole afternoon, her tape recorder reeling, and I was juiced at the thought of expressing myself to what was at least a tributary of the mainstream. I was full of insufferable opinions, I fear, grand and glam and playing to the balcony. What appeared about two months later was a two-page profile called "Proust on the Pacific," the most excruciating aspect of which was that the title was a direct quotation. I argued that the mythic realm of Hollywood was ripe for a troubadour (me) who would seize its jeweled heart. I sounded like . . . well, Norma Scoop herself, overblown and blowsy and insufferably precious.

Around that time, 1979 or thereabouts, I was in San Francisco to give a reading at the oldest (indeed, the only) gay and lesbian bookstore in the Bay Area. I spent an evening with an old friend from the Boston years, a writer who was in residence at a local university. He was living in a latter-day hippie commune with a half dozen other bohemian types. Amid much laughter my friend and I went off to dinner, accompanied by the young man who rented the attic room.

A quiet-spoken, self-effacing sort, who did manage to tell me he was a stringer for one of the gay rags. All evening I thought he and my friend were an item, but I was too Waspy polite to ask them directly. I had never experienced the particular press negotiation as to what was "on the record" and what was off. *I* didn't think we were having an interview. The dish flew fast and loose as I regaled them with tales out of school about Hollywood movers and shakers. We were all entertaining one another, I thought, with no holds barred when it came to being outrageous.

On Sunday I returned to L.A., told Roger about our friend's peregrinations in academia, and never even mentioned the tyro journalist. Ten days later the bookstore owner in San Francisco sent me a clipping from one of the alternative weeklies. The meek-mannered tyro had done me up as a feature, regaling his audience with nuggets about this glib and fatuous lightweight from Tinseltown. He repeated stories about the mating habits of stars that were never meant to go beyond the hair dryer. He painted me as a rich son-of-a-bitch, pulling zeroes out of the air as he speculated about my unearned income.

I'd talked too much, it was as simple as that. No excuse not to have realized that a journalist, however much a dweeb in person, was always taking notes for a story. And if I was too stupid to specify *off the record,* then he could hardly be blamed for assuming every word I said was *on*—fair game, as it were. I'd forgotten the first rule of caution, most tellingly expressed in Joan Didion's preface to *Slouching Towards Bethlehem:*

> My only advantage as a reporter is that I am so physically small, so temperamentally unobtrusive, and so neurotically inarticulate that people tend to forget that my presence runs counter to their best interests. And it always does. That is one last thing to remember: *writers are always selling somebody out.*[1]

---

1. Joan Didion, *Slouching Towards Bethlehem* (New York: Farrar, Straus & Giroux, 1968), page xvi.

My comings and goings went pretty much unreported during the next few years, when I was working as a bottom-feeder in the Hollywood sewer system. At that time anyway, writers were the very last players in the fame game. Yet even then I managed to score a few points, though I hadn't hit the ball myself, hadn't so much as taken a swing. I had just turned in a screenplay to Universal, my first for hire. In other words, I'd launched myself into a system which would tear the pages into confetti, and the confetti into dust. All of that would take a couple of years, the inchmeal cure for innocence.

But in the first flush of studiochat, some enterprising publicist had leaked a blind item. I woke up one morning to find myself, picture and all, in Liz Smith's column in the *Daily News*. The caption under my beamish face was this: *From zilch to $150,000.* The accompanying story told of my meteoric rise to the heights of lucre, so sizzling was my screenplay. Not a word of it true, but so what? It upped the ante of interest among those bankable stars who could get a picture greenlighted. And thus ensued a period of delirious fallout, during which Dustin and Meryl and Faye and Warren were variously bandied about as "this close" to a deal.

Don't hold your breath. My screenplay would be lining birdcages soon enough. But for *years* afterward I would hear from marginal forgotten friends and guys I went to college with. They'd seen my Liz Smith item in syndication in the morning paper, from Baltimore to Singapore. I was congratulated a good deal more for the item than for the screenplay — which by then had long faded into development limbo, land of the undead. The prevailing sound bite about me, whether I liked it or not, was that I was rich and famous. Well, I didn't mind it that much. But it struck me even at the time that the press could paint an image of you without any input from you at all. And without any countervailing influence, that image took hold as the truth.

I could see why actors and other royals went ballistic when

they read the lies and slander perpetrated by the tabloid press. At the same time I could see what an easy ride they had from the mainstream Hollywood press, where the news was always soft and cutesy. A true collaboration of press-agentry and a willing mouthpiece, oiled by princely lunches and floral tributes so lush that a journalist had to paw his way through orchids to get to his computer. Good publicity was all. And of course they wouldn't dream of mentioning that anyone was gay or lesbian. The show marriages were enshrined like the spun-sugar figures crowning a wedding cake. No one ever bothered to report that the cake was made of Eisenhower's snots.

Cut to 1988, when I published *Borrowed Time*. By then I had been in the AIDS trenches for a good five years, and my main perception of the press was nauseated contempt for their non-coverage of the calamity. To be sure, there had been an avalanche of stories surrounding the death of Rock Hudson in the fall of '85. But their main thrust was prurient, with a scarcely concealed overlay of *Schadenfreude*. And of course they affected to be "shocked, shocked"—in the immortal words of Claude Rains in *Casablanca*—to learn that Hudson was gay.

Make no mistake, the press was as much to blame as the Reagan/Bush genocide machine for the gloating ignorance and shame that attached to this "gay disease." Their constitutional inability to talk about gay in any context at all—the editors were men's men—precluded even a pretense of compassion. When I agreed to go out on the road with *Borrowed Time,* an eight-city tour, I was wary at best, frightened at worst. Already there had been reports of camera crews refusing to be in the same studio as a person with AIDS. The country was in full-scale panic, no amount of reassurance convincing the populace that the virus couldn't be passed by mosquito and toilet seat.

I went first to Houston, my virgin exposure to drive-time call-ins. Sitting across from the host in flyboy earphones, scarcely exchanging a word with him as he zigzagged from ad spot to weather to Debbie June in the traffic chopper. He had clearly never so much as opened my book, relying on the poop sheet from the publisher. "You look all right to me," he said. "How much time do you think you have?" He seemed concerned that I might go into a coma right there in his sound booth. Always in those years one had to begin with AIDS 101, countering the stupefying lack of information. And when we turned it over to the phones, the first caller informed me that I had got exactly what I deserved, almost gleeful that the nation would soon be rid of the whole lot of us Sodomites.

That was the general tone in the summer of '88. In Berkeley, on the Pacifica station, which tended to have a liberal/rad listenership, a woman told me that she'd read in a book passed out in church that "you homosexamils eat each other's feces because you've got the devil inside you." I'd never given much thought, frankly, to the devil's diet. But I was beginning to get a grip on slinging the shit right back—ticking off the dangerous lunacies of the Christian fundies and their loving dictum that we should all "Thank God for AIDS."

In Boston, a caller to WBZ Radio earnestly demanded that everyone with AIDS be quarantined. And how were we going to do that? "All those Jap barracks in California," he replied instantly. "That'd be perfect. Or send all these sickos to live with the Indians, and blockade all the roads."

"Sir," I replied dryly, "do you know what a concentration camp is?"

"You're damn right I do. It's time we started building them again, too."

That tour was my first encounter with raw hate, and what was so chilling about it was how nationwide its reach was. On the whole the radio hosts didn't challenge any of the lies, leaving it to me to extricate myself as best I could. By comparison, the print media were a saner class entirely. Over and over I'd sit down with mainstream reporters, quickly aware of how

many were coming from a place of pain and shame. If they
didn't apologize directly for their papers' sins of omission in
covering the plague, they would almost always blurt out that
their brother or neighbor or high school sweetheart had died
of AIDS. They were determined to right the balance, to clear
their own conscience if nothing else.

I didn't set out to be the AIDS Poster Boy, but willingly
entered the breach in cities that hadn't yet put a face to the
epidemic. Rock Hudson and Ryan White were not enough,
too easily dismissed with a curt *Not me* on the way to the
sports page. There were hundreds of cases all around, but none
with sufficient access to the media. In many places I was the
first feature profile, certainly the first taste of nuclear rage as I
ticked off the culprits at the NIH and the CDC.

Generally, these encounters with the press were a nice curative for the drive-time citizen hate squad. Not that even the
most passionate and well-meaning of them could keep up with
the gay and lesbian press, which had been covering the horrors
of the war since the first cases surfaced in '81. Our own reporters had grown leaner and tougher in the heat of battle, and
they'd developed a rigorous skepticism about the numbers put
out by the government. For ten years we were asked to believe
that the infected HIV population in the States was a cool million. Never a change in that statistic, even as the full-blown
caseload climbed above the quarter million mark. It was as if
the epidemic had stopped in its tracks to allow a head count,
and from then on a million was the benchmark—and such a
nice round number besides, so why revise it? To admit that
the numbers kept growing and growing would have made
them have to face the burgeoning caseload of women and adolescents.

The mainstream press, like so many sheep, accepted whatever the government said. It was journalism by press release.
Whereas the gay and lesbian journalists knew how to call a lie

a lie and made mincemeat of the bureaucrats' every pro-
nouncement. The New York *Native* probably led the way,
questioning the validity of HIV itself, accusing the establishment of fudging the basic science. Their hectoring campaign
against AZT bordered on the nutty, to be sure, yet time is
beginning to prove them close to the mark. Then, they were
prophets without honor in a system ruled by drug conglomerates and Reagan's Mormon appointees.

And even as we covered the story better, withering all the
government's forays in spin control, that group of writers who
had colonized the margin after Stonewall had grown into a
juggernaut of personal witness. Andrew Holleran was writing
knife-edge essays for *Christopher Street,* pulling them together
in *Ground Zero.* Ed White and Adam Mars-Jones had collabo-
rated on a collection of stories— *The Darker Proof*—alternating
voices of the damned. Larry Kramer, our very own Cassandra,
had written a devastating indictment of complacency, "1112
and Counting," and followed it up with the white-hot Brecht-
ian fury of *The Normal Heart.*

Witnessing was for most of us a way to keep from going
mad. In city after city, the most provincial of which now supported a vital gay and lesbian bookstore, I'd face a line of war-
torn refugees who wanted their books inscribed. *My lover died
last week,* one would tell me; and the next, a woman who
couldn't stop crying, would choke out that she'd lost two
brothers in a single year. Nurses who worked in AIDS wards;
the children of secret bisexuals, still in shellshock. And the sick
themselves, bone-thin and limping from neuropathy, pared
down to the last essential core, refined by fire until they
seemed as pure as crystal, waiting to shatter. Besides being unbearably moving, they came to honor me for my writing—till
I thought I would shatter myself out of sheer unworthiness.

But as far as *all the news that's fit to print* was concerned, it
was all taking place in a faraway country, remote as the cloud

of flies that swarmed about the starving in the Sudan. Good for the occasional wrenching update, but not the least bit sexy. *And we were that country.* Dying in the corridors of emergency rooms because body bags were easier to fill than beds. Burnout was the general rule among those who'd stayed too long at the front, and the geometric numbers led to what they called *multiple loss syndrome.* So now we had two syndromes going at once, the sickness unto death and the emptiness after, like juggling a pair of chainsaws. And no one gave a damn unless we did, shouting into the din of indifference, in George Whitmore's haunting phrase: *Someone was here.*

I didn't go out on the road again for another two years. I gave a few incendiary speeches, and in October '88 took part in the exorcism of the FDA, working with Vito Russo as press liaison, copping a millisecond of national exposure on the *CBS Evening News.* I started getting called for sound bites by reporters on the AIDS beat, especially to comment on the latest cure-of-the-week. I tried to take my cue from Larry Kramer, spouting a whole laundry list of the closeted creeps who kept letting us die. If I didn't develop quite the reputation as a crank that Larry did, it was not for want of trying. I hammered at the televangelist queens and their brain-dead flocks, and announced that I no longer considered myself an American. Reagan/Bush had erased my citizenship.

By then the press and the country at large had found themselves a safe and tangible focus for the epidemic: the Quilt. It gave them permission to grieve and to wonder at the vastness of what was already lost. I wouldn't dream of diminishing the heart's force and anguish that stitched every patch of that monument. It resonated with healing power, bringing together legions of those left behind, heretofore isolated in scarred home towns and decimated cities. The Quilt shone with human endurance and the deepest family feeling. Wherever it went the minicam vans were there, close-up on brokenhearted remnants as the beat reporter provided voiceover in sepulchral tones.

But I also understand why Steve, who'd sewn his share of panels over the years, would fly into a rage as the end approached: "And don't put me in that fucking quilt!" Being of a mind to have his body dumped instead on the White House lawn. The Quilt had begun to seem too passive, even too nice, letting the war criminals off the hook and providing the media with far too easy a wrapup. Much neater than trying to unravel the Gordian knot of AIDS activism, the Byzantine infighting and turf protection, the in-your-face bad manners of those who wouldn't go quietly. The quilted dead made for prettier sound bites, especially effective at zeroing in on the "innocent" victims, the kids and the hemophiliacs.

At the same time there began to appear a certain overview phenomenon under the general rubric of AIDS-and-the-Arts. Typically these were hand-wringing accounts of the impact of so much cultured dying, lamenting for instance the White Way silence left by Michael Bennett, the songs unsung. This litany was something of a mixed bag, bringing under the same umbrella the likes of Way Bandy and Halston, Miss Kitty and Keith Haring. Though it was surely true what Fran Lebowitz had so scathingly observed—

> If you removed all of the homosexuals and homosexual influence from what is generally regarded as American culture, you would be pretty much left with "Let's Make a Deal."

—these roundups of the arts tended to foster in the general populace ever new heights of *Not me*.

As if artists breathed too rarefied an air, had far too much sex for their own good, and were generally frail from living on coffee and cigarettes. Reminiscent of Susan Sontag's isolation of the consumptive personality in *Illness as Metaphor,* the Camille/Keats temperament, which served to distance a previous century from the country of the diseased.

Not that these various paeans to the disappeared among the artists weren't well-meaning. But they tended to conveniently not notice how many of the creative folk died with a lie on their lips, the death certificate as a kind of final cover-up. Died of lymphoma, died of a staph infection, anything but AIDS. The media couldn't seem to make the connection between the silencing by death and the Neanderthal backlash against the likes of Robert Mapplethorpe and David Wojnarowich. There was mad rejoicing among the Philistines and the family-values thugs about the double good fortune of snuffing out fags and dangerous artists in one fell swoop.

The hand-wringing reached a sort of apogee of sentimental dithering in the *Newsweek* cover story on the death of Rudolph Nureyev. While they strewed the bier with violets, eliciting prayerful reminiscences, Nureyev's doctor in Paris was rigorously denying rumors that the dancer had succumbed to AIDS. That was the final straw for this camel's back. Twelve years of fighting to tear down the prison of shame, to give the stricken some dignity, and this *prima ballerina* had singlehandedly restored to AIDS the status of dirty little secret.

I didn't question anyone's desire to keep his illness private. But to keep up appearances *after* death, especially for such an international figure, simply would not do. "I don't care how great a dancer he was," I told *Newsweek.* "He died a coward." This was not especially a popular sentiment at the time, but for my whole adult life I'd been hearing Nureyev pooh-pooh that he was gay. It was as if he lived in the high empyrean of the Muses, *hors de catégorie,* way above the tacky politics of gay. As *Vanity Fair* was quick to dish, this did not prevent him from cruising the parks and watering holes of queer Manhattan by night. So in denial about his own illness that he consistently rejected his diagnosis to his doctor's face. And never a penny, so far as anyone knew, to a single gay and lesbian cause. But thanks for the pirouettes anyway.

I won't pretend that my burst of outrage had any effect on the doctor's decision to take back the lie, owning up to AIDS at a second news conference a few days later. He may well have realized on his own what a grotesque distortion his cover-up represented, how dismissive of the sufferings of millions. What I did manage to achieve, however, was the status of full-fledged crank—especially among balletomanes.

But here I am getting ahead of myself. I went out on the road again in the spring of 1990, this time with a novel to hawk. It was fairly quickly obvious that the press was inclined to be more sympathetic, if no bolder. A couple of print reporters who'd interviewed me the last time around had died in the interim, and not of old age. Several others actually pleaded with me to give them some new angle—any new angle— since their editors and bosses had decided that AIDS was yesterday's news.

I rose to the task immediately, sketching a portrait of the AIDS underground and its traffic in non–FDA-approved drugs. I was still pushing the fairy-tale notion that a regimen of effective medication was imminent—a mix of antivirals and immune boosters, what we called "the cocktail." Yet even as those drugs became available, I cautioned, they'd be out of reach of America's vast Third World of poverty, where the virus burned like an inferno. I gave ACT UP a plug wherever possible, countering mistrust that we activists had gone too far this time. *What would YOU do,* I'd ask, *if you knew they had the drugs that would give you another year but refused to release them?*

Perhaps I had an easier time of it because the publisher had carefully avoided booking most of the drive-time call-in market. Or at least I was lucky to be playing the high end, Sonya Friedman on CNN and several appearances on Michael

Jackson's brainy show on ABC Talk Radio. When I reached
Chicago I thought there had been some mixup, for I was
scheduled to go on the air with a veteran right-wing smoothie
who didn't bother to hide his upright Mormonism or his loyalty to Reagan/Bush. The publicist in New York knew only
that the guy had asked for me, promising to treat me and my
social diseases with a little respect. Deep down I figured he'd
probably ambush me, but I wasn't afraid of a shouting match
if it came to that.

I was ushered into the sound booth, two minutes to air-
time, just as he was finishing sports. They went to commercial,
and he shook my hand. A red-faced man in his sixties, bags
under his eyes like steamer trunks and having a nuclear bad-
hair-day. He told me he was sorry for all my losses and apologized for not reading my book. "I'm not going to take any
callers," he said carefully. "My audience isn't exactly on your
side." Whichever way he liked, I retorted. "Ten seconds,
Ray," the producer bleeped in. But Ray was still taking his
time, his basset face sagging with pain, looking away as he
finally blurted it out. "I just found out—I mean he told me—
my son is a homosexual. Good kid. I guess I've had it all
wrong."

And we were on. His voice took on a craggy upbeat tone,
avuncular and cozy, as he warned his audience not to change
the station. I understood that what he'd told me was off-the-
record, and that I'd heard all he was going to tell me. In the
on-air segment he treated me with kid gloves, letting me make
an impassioned plea for tolerance and complain that we'd
wasted a decade scapegoating AIDS. He thanked me and went
to commercial again. My publicist/driver bustled in to whisk
me away, leaving me scarcely a moment to shake Ray's hand.
"Your son's a lucky man," I said, and then both of us turned
away.

All through Washington, Philadelphia, and New York I

couldn't get it out of my mind. Did he understand that I meant the boy was lucky to have him as a father? Didn't his Mormon bylaws require that the kid be shunned, his name unchiseled from the stone mountain of the blessed forever? Was he just gay, or did he have AIDS? I can still see the grappling in his father's eyes, the shaken faith. But more than anything else I saw the transfiguring power of a truth that had finally hit home. For better or worse, Mormon-wise, Ray was on our side now.

In New York we had managed to set up an appearance on *Geraldo,* and I agreed to be on the panel as long as Larry Kramer would join me. Talk about a venue where no respectable poet had gone before. Media-savvy friends warned me I was heading into quicksand, a tabloid format that managed to cheapen everything it touched. But I couldn't pass up a chance to address so large an audience, especially if they weren't the sort that ever read books. And the actual experience proved to be wholly satisfying, not least because Geraldo Rivera himself was superbly informed. He'd read the books and understood the numbers, and was using the occasion in a conscious effort to elevate the debate among his viewers.

Larry and I fell naturally into good cop/bad cop mode. Larry held up a sign accusing the writer on the plague desk of *The New York Times* of being "the worst AIDS reporter in America." We'd both been doing it so long that we were able to bulletin the tragedies and crimes of the epidemic rapid-fire, scarcely pausing for breath. I was the widow, reeling off the unimaginable pain and grief of families and lovers. One of our panelists was a lachrymose TV reporter from San Francisco, clearly very far gone himself. We left it to him to cover the dying part. And poor Mary McFadden, there to represent the design industry's commitment to stopping AIDS. When she proudly announced that they hoped to raise a million at some event, Larry turned on her in high dudgeon. Million shmillion. Calvin Klein could write a check that big himself and not even miss it. Larry was especially hard on the self-satisfaction of charities. McFadden scarcely uttered another peep.

It was the AIDS circus in miniature. All that was needed to complete the circle was an official government liar and a peabrained televangelist. But I left that Times Square studio in a state of real exhilaration, figuring we had mixed it up in a way that showed how Hydra-headed was the monster we were fighting. And the upshot was that for *weeks* after the show aired, strangers would come up to me in the street, in coffee shops and multiplexes, to shake my hand and tell me they had seen me on *Geraldo*. Flattering in a surreal way, and meant to show support for my personal battle. But I was hard put to understand how so much individual decency would ever translate into public policy, however many minds we managed to change.

Over the next months I found it harder and harder to get it up for a one-man show of defiance and tempered optimism. I'd written four books about AIDS, and began to despair that a hundred books like *Borrowed Time* couldn't seem to save a single life. A period of diminishing returns, which ended up leaving me feeling both useless and used. I received plaques and proclamations from various organizations, glad to do it if it helped raise money to ease the dying. But I started to feel like a monument before my time, already stuck in a niche. And then Steve died at the end of the summer, not a month after I'd finished writing a love story whose joy was all because of him.

Sometime that autumn I heard that Larry was telling the press and our so-called leaders that the AIDS war was over and we'd lost it. That expressed it best, it seemed to me. Those magic bullets we'd smuggled in from Thailand and China and Mexico and France had all proven to be duds. The scientists bickered, and the politicians slashed. Nothing was going to stop the deaths of hundreds of thousands more gay men before this beast was brought under control. And as salt in the wound, new studies were reporting that younger gay men weren't practicing safer sex anymore. Who cared, after all?

And yet, like a trained seal, I went out on tour again in the summer of '91, happily with Winston at my side. I talked about the novel I'd written for Steve, and what it meant to fall in love in the midst of war. AIDS was an absolute fact of life by then, intractable as poverty, no new angles and not much hope except among the New Age happy talkers. It was all I could do to speak about the difficulty of love in a race with time. I got about as much coverage as any other AIDS institution—a certain *pro forma* respect, lip service to the notion that two men could love as wholly as anyone else. As to how grotesque it was to bury two lovers and know that a third would bury me—that was a bit too much for the lifestyle pages.

By the time I took the dog-and-pony show out for *Becoming a Man,* I was six months into my own diagnosis, having nearly bought the farm with a drug reaction over New Year's. Two months later I had my first KS lesions, on my shoulder blade and the roof of my mouth. In June I was in for toxo, forcing me to cancel the East Coast leg of the tour, but somehow pulling it together in time for the western leg. By then the only occasions that meant anything to me were the bookstore signings, especially the queer ones. You knew that whoever showed up didn't need AIDS 101, and they seemed as ready as I to talk about something else for a change. In this case, the suffocation of the closet and the struggle to free ourselves from the last vestiges of self-hatred.

That ought to have been my swan song as a public figure in the flesh—though admittedly the last five years were beginning to resemble the farewell tour of an aging mezzo-soprano, milking those high notes for all they were worth. But I hadn't counted on the nomination for the National Book Award. Thus we found ourselves in tuxes, Winston and I, in the solid gold ballroom of the Plaza. Sitting around a table with my editor, agent, and publicist, as well as the Joint Chiefs of Harcourt Brace. Having sternly announced to everyone I knew that I didn't stand an iceberg's chance in hell of winning.

Be careful what you don't dare wish for. When they announced my name the table fairly levitated in shocked delight, and the next five minutes were practically an out-of-body experience as I made my way to the judges' dais. All the Oscar speeches I'd made in my pajamas since I was eight—or kneeling before the King in Stockholm—happily didn't fail me. Like Maureen Stapleton I had the urge to thank everyone I'd ever met.

But I never did get back to my veal scallopini. With barely a segue I was in the middle of a press conference, grinning ear to ear as I answered the questions they lobbed at me, not a spitball in the bunch. I only recall them asking if I was the first gay writer to cop the prize. Probably not, I replied, but certainly the first person with AIDS. Of course I could've talked all night, but they had deadlines to meet. And it was time to yield the mike to Mary Oliver, who'd won the prize in poetry for an unsparing body of work—the smell of skunk in the morning air, the "old woman made out of leaves." In her own acceptance speech she'd paid tribute to her lover, so the story of these awards was a gay and lesbian story, one way or another.

The avalanche of press attention would continue from mid-November to Christmas. Camera crews tracked heavy cable through the house, sending the dogs for cover. The print photographers had me frozen in various pretzel poses for hours at a stretch. But what was not to like about so much attention? The level of intelligence was gratifying in the extreme. They weren't too timid to include the dying part, and yet managed not to exploit it either. If this was my swan song with the press, it was easy as eating ice cream. All the same, by New Year's I was weary of it—time to go back to my essays and this race against the clock.

I had my moments of comeuppance, to be sure. A friend from Boston had left an impish message to the effect that now I had my Oscar for *Butterfield 8*—a reference to the prize they withheld from Elizabeth Taylor for *Cat on a Hot Tin Roof,* and the sympathy vote that put her over two years later in homage to her tracheotomy. The implication was that the powers that be in bookdom were making up for *Borrowed Time.* In some quarters there were dark rumblings that the judges had bowed to Political Correctness—though one of their number assured me at the ceremony that PC had worked against me first to last.

In any case, lest I be getting a swelled head from so much attention, I could always bring myself down a peg by recalling the *People* interview. During which I expatiated at length about the Greeks and the river of wisdom that coursed through all the centuries. When I finally paused for breath after fifteen minutes of loftiness, the interviewer grabbed his chance to ask the overriding question: "Who does the cooking?"

II

Bear with me now—I have to backtrack to September '91. I'd finished the draft of *Becoming a Man* on Labor Day, seventeen years to the day after I met Roger. Winston and I were scheduled to leave for New York in mid-September, where I would attend two days of meetings at WNET, preliminary to writing a script about a multicultural cross-section of people with AIDS who are brought together in a drug study. We planned to drive up to Provincetown afterward, ·for a weekend on the cusp of autumn. Before we left I spent a few days answering a pile of mail from my readers, the old Wasp etiquette rearing its head: no letter must go unacknowledged.

An unusual missive had arrived that very week, written on lined paper in a kid's most earnest penmanship. His name was Tony Johnson, age thirteen, and he was writing to commend me for *Borrowed Time* and *Love Alone*. Apologizing that he hadn't actually bought them, but traded them with a guy in the hospital for a stack of sports magazines. He didn't have AIDS, he told me, but understood about pain and chronic illness from his own experience. Parenthetically almost, he revealed that he'd been physically abused for years by his birth parents, hastening to add that he'd been adopted since by wonderful people. No self-pity, and especially no wish to bother me.

I sent a reply, just one of a couple of dozen, wishing Tony Johnson well and telling him he probably had the distinction of being my youngest fan. Ten days later we were back from our East Coast jaunt, and I discovered a message on my machine from Tony's adoptive mother—I'll call her Gayle. She said my note had really given him a boost, especially as his health just then was very rocky. She asked nothing from me either, but on impulse I picked up the phone and called. I coaxed from her the details of the boy's punishing journey— the sex abuse by his parents and their friends, serving him up like a sacrificial lamb for the sake of their darkest pleasures. Virtual starvation. And constant savage beatings, such that when he finally escaped the horror, the x-rays showed fifty-four bones broken throughout his riddled body.

As I would later say in my foreword to Tony's book, all I wanted to do right then was run. I'd been through enough torment and meaningless tragedy for close to a decade, and the last thing I needed was another case assignment. Gayle could hear the flinching in my voice and hastened to reassure me: "You don't *have* to talk to him. But you'll like him, I promise. He's not depressing at all."

Well, all right. And a half-minute later he was on the line, shy at first or a little in awe, but with an overriding hunger to talk to someone who understood. Now I have to say how cautious I was in these matters, having heard a veritable Homeric catalogue of miseries in the previous few years, as readers reached out to connect. I drew a certain line in the sand, answering a letter once but almost never writing a second time to the same correspondent. I couldn't serve as everyone's support group; couldn't begin to slog through the piles of manuscripts that arrived every week, written in blood and tears. Besides, I wasn't in the market for any new friends. Even if most of my own friends were ghosts now, they were still the only ones who really understood *me*—as opposed to the Paul Monette who wrote my books. Otherwise I had Winston and the dogs and Victor, and that was about the limit of my heart's capacity. And I need to add that I'd never been especially good with kids, old as I was before my time, old by the time I was ten in fact. I never quite got the hang of them as a species.

But this kid was so disarming, so ebullient, loved to laugh so much, that I made an exception and found him room in the inner circle. It probably had a lot to do with the imminence of our two diagnoses. Tony might not have AIDS officially, but I for one wasn't buying that. When they first brought him in he had second-stage syphilis; and he'd suffered a stroke since then, having to learn to walk all over again. He was subject to "bleeds," which sounded like spontaneous eruptions from the magma of his tainted blood.

I got into the habit of calling him late at night, after Winston had gone to bed, because I knew they only slept in snatches in Tony's house. I got to know "the body mechanic," as Tony called him—a doctor friend who'd moved into the Johnson household for the duration, bearing the kid to the emergency room sometimes three and four times a week. Gayle's husband had meanwhile been called up from the Reserves and was mostly incommunicado. Tony would talk for hours about how lucky he'd been to land in such a loving home, where he actually had his own room, the first bed he'd ever slept in. A pair of sisters came with the deal, who bragged about having such a supersmart big brother. Indeed, he was exceedingly bright, finishing high school with tutors before he was thirteen. We'd talk until the grate came clanking down, announcing that the bar across the street had closed for the night. It meant to Tony Johnson that he'd made it through another day.

Then, it must've been a month later, he finally broke through with an AIDS infection—no news to anybody in his inner circle, though the family were devastated all the same. I said all the appropriate hollow things, but at least convinced Tony that now we were "moonmen" together, refering to the exile Roger and I had felt in *Borrowed Time*. Mostly to distract him, I proposed with his permission to use him as the model for a character in *Trials*. He eagerly accepted, demanding copies of every outline and memo, then every scene direct from the computer. He was the one who helped *me,* if you want to know the truth, not the other way around. When he confided that he'd always wanted to write himself—an ambition second only to being inducted into the Baseball Hall of Fame—I encouraged him to start keeping a journal. The least he'd be able to do was leave something behind for the people who loved him. Who knew how many others he might help?

He was skeptical and uncertain, too sick most of the time to hold a pen. He'd already lost the sight in one eye, and during the next several months would be diagnosed with TB and lose a leg to lymphoma. They were living in quarantine now. Tony was on the losing end so much that he could hardly keep track of it all. Happily, one of his growing circle of lifeline friends—which now included Mister Rogers from the TV Neighborhood—had the foresight to contact the Make-a-Wish Foundation on Tony's behalf.

After all the paperwork was done, all the doctors' signatures concurring that the boy was on his way out, the Foundation came through with a computer. Tony got so wrapped up in it that in a matter of weeks he could practically get the machine to make peanut-butter sandwiches—whereas I have always compared my own ten years' progress with computer technology to teaching a slow monkey how to tell time.

Throughout most of the winter and spring of '92 he worked like a demon, instinctively discovering a form for himself in the short personal essay. Tales of life on the meanest streets, filtered through the strays and throwaway children who constituted his outer world. What was so unusual right from the start was a rare consistency of tone, at once plucky and philosophical, racing against his own clock to try to figure out what it all meant. But here again, no self-pity, so that when he waxed sentimental he'd earned it. Somehow he had survived his tormentors with his heart intact, and he had a gift for the quick study of character, the *David Copperfield* eccentrics who crossed his path. As his battle with AIDS intensified, he saw the rank intolerance and dehumanization that went with it, refusing to be seen as an "innocent" victim. He had a lot to say about prejudice.

Not that every insight didn't come with a struggle, for he had to husband all his strength to get through the 106° fevers and the treatments to drain his lungs, a surgical procedure performed without anesthetic. Nurses would grab the toys he'd brought from home and toss them in with the infectious waste. Doctors would leaf through his chart and irritably inquire, "Isn't this kid dead yet?" Just loud enough for the kid to hear.

Swamped as I was myself by then with the tortures of the medically damned, it was all I could do to hold onto a couple of hours a day to write *Trials*. Our check-in calls to one another grew more infrequent, though Tony would always call when he had a new piece finished. He read each one over the phone, in that pre-adolescent voice that stubbornly refused to deepen—the only thing among all his troubles that seemed to bruise his vanity. At the end of every recital I'd tell him what a good job he was doing, but now go on to the next one. No time to bask in it yet.

When at last he had a presentable manuscript I told him I would send it along to my agent, Wendy Weil. But I cautioned him not to get too invested in publication, because the market forces were out of our hands. I was hard put myself to figure who the audience was, and certainly hadn't a clue how the Young Adult sector worked. In any case, I knew I was far too close to his work to judge its merits. Fortuitously, Wendy responded with enthusiasm, submitting the manuscript to David Groff, my editor at Crown. And after an agonizing interval, building support in-house, David came back and said yes. Amidst the ensuing blizzard of contracts and revisions, I consciously pulled back, allowing Tony the full measure of an experience he'd hardly dared to dream. He turned out to be quite a skilled negotiator, actually, absorbing the arcana of the system as quickly as he did the rest of the world, with a street kid's smarts.

Of course I was thrilled for him, proud as a stepfather once removed. Sometimes after all, it seemed, there were motions of grace in the fallen world. Yet I couldn't imagine how he'd ever survive long enough to see it in print. On the hustings last summer with *Becoming a Man,* I referred to Tony often, especially as an example to illustrate the glass walls of the pharmaceutical cabal. What had saved my brain from toxo that very month was a new drug, still experimental, which was also a good last-ditch treatment for the AIDS pneumonia. And yet, though Tony's lungs were in shreds by then, he proved ineligible for "compassionate use" because he was too young or didn't weigh enough or some other idiotic Catch-22.

Whenever Winston and I were in New York, of course, Gayle would ask us to come visit Tony. But I was too scared of being exposed to TB, no amount of reassurance quite convincing me that all I'd need was a mask and gown. I did write a foreword for the book, however, now officially titled *A Rock and a Hard Place.* By that point I was deep into my own volume of essays, and didn't doubt that Tony's example had helped to crystallize the form for me. Perhaps it's I who don't exist, and Tony Johnson's the ghostwriter.

His book was scheduled for publication in April of '93. I didn't have any input with Crown's publicity engine, though I understood Gayle's passion to protect the boy's privacy. Of course he couldn't go out on the road, couldn't even leave his oxygen tent. Gayle agreed to let him be interviewed by telephone, unless it took too much out of him. He couldn't have his picture published because there were still people out there who could retaliate, criminals who'd abused him. Tony was understandably terrified about any further contact with the source of all his nightmares. This wasn't just paranoia on the Johnsons' part; but even if it had been, I didn't blame Gayle for standing firm.

In February I was diagnosed with CMV retinitis and had to submit to a daily IV drip. I was also going to radiology five times a week, to try to zap the swelling in my leg. My brain was beginning to misfire again, despite the new drug. For a while I pulled back from a good deal more than Tony, sick of giving status reports on the breakdown of my mortal flesh, frightened that the juggle of meds and treatments was starting to feel unacceptable.

Even so, I followed Tony's literary progress. Generous quotes had come in from the likes of Bernie Siegel, the wellness guru, and Marva Collins, distinguished advocate for children and founder of Westside Prep. The movie rights were grabbed up by Lorimar while the book was still in galleys. With that windfall Tony bought himself a jukebox. The early reviews in the trade publications were excellent, and the book-chat press seemed comfortable with the rules laid down by the publisher—no pictures, no face-to-face, all interviews by telephone. The only advice I remember giving Tony at the outset was the Didion caution: journalists aren't your friends, however cozily they may present themselves.

A reporter for the Associated Press, Leslie Dreyfous, sent

out on the wire a sympathetic story that ran in several papers across the country. A poignant feature about Tony appeared in *USA Today*. He made a phone appearance on one of the afternoon talk shows in New York. He was already receiving mail from other abused kids, applauding his courage and example. A teacher in Pennsylvania wanted to use the book in her middle school health classes. Winston said he was going to sell more books than all of mine put together.

But at the same time, gremlins began to rear their heads. In the Midwest, a self-important booby who called himself a doctor (which in fact he wasn't) took it upon himself to mount a one-man disinformation campaign, calling up reporters at *The New York Times, The Wall Street Journal, USA Today,* and the Associated Press. He contended that no fourteen-year-old could have possibly written such a sophisticated book as *A Rock and a Hard Place.* There was clearly no Tony Johnson at all, but the booby had figured out the scam. The actual author of this meretricious book was Paul Monette, a homosexual writer whose own work about AIDS had failed to garner sympathy from the straight world. Therefore I had made up a pediatric case to get attention for the cause—which of course was that old right-wing bugbear, the homosexual agenda.

The first word I had of it came from a reporter at *The New York Times.* She asked me if this slander bore any truth at all, and when I said no, she warned me there was a troublemaker out there who wanted my scalp. He had pestered Crown for proof that Tony existed and had been rebuffed. It only made him more fanatical, as he contacted reporters who'd written stories about Tony and demanded they expose this fraud. I wasn't too concerned about it, wondering idly if I'd drawn the vengeful wrath of some balletomane. But from the snippets that reached my ears, I began to suspect we were dealing with a Christian fundie. They can't bear that the truth be told about child abuse, because they're at the top of the list of perpetrators. The Bible *tells* them to beat their kids.

Thus flippantly did I ignore the rising slime. I was stable again, and had just finished "Mustering" in the latter part of May. Then, one Saturday afternoon, I had an ashen call from David Groff, who told me *Newsweek* was going to press on Monday with a story that Tony didn't exist and I was the ghostly author. David hadn't yet seen the story himself but expected to have it in hand by nightfall. In the intervening hours I thought first about poor Tony, who'd spilled his guts to tell the hard truth, only to have it dismissed as a fairy tale. And I of course was the fairy in question. Backed into a corner by innuendo, forced to issue denials, a classic no-win case of *Do you still beat your wife?*

Then David called back and read me the full allegation. Under the title "The Author Nobody's Met," the reporter triumphantly detailed the results of her personal sleuthing— *Nancy Drew and the Missing Wunderkind.* The burden of it was that none of us had ever met Tony Johnson in the flesh—not me, not David, not Wendy, not Mister Rogers, not Make-a-Wish. We were all being deluded by a telephone voice, "a soprano that could belong to a woman as convincingly as to a boy." I'd been talking to this boy two or three times a week for almost two years; it was dumbfounding to hear it all reduced to the level of a cheap thriller. And the tone of the piece? Mocking and sardonic: "Trying to find the real Tony is like getting trapped in a page of *Where's Waldo?*"

It was two days before I had the magazine in hand, so the full-bore tabloid breathlessness didn't hit me until then. But Nancy Drew, in her mind anyway, was clearly on the trail of a Pulitzer:

Who's the author behind Tony? One possibility is Monette, 47, whose moving works about AIDS Tony seems to mimic and who declared in a *New York Times* interview last year, "I've become a very political creature." He couldn't be reached [they never tried], but

> Weil, his agent, denies Monette scripted Tony. Still,
> both know baseball and books. Both find themselves
> in Connecticut. Both loathe book reports and love
> plush afghans.

It was ludicrous. So fiercely do I detest the National Pastime
that one of my strongest memories of growing up is fleeing
the house at the mere sound of a baseball game on the radio.
Baseball represents to me all the hetero torment of being
forced to be "normal."

But how do you issue that kind of denial? Obviously
Nancy Drew had only looked at one book of mine — *Halfway
Home,* a novel about two brothers, one gay and one straight,
whose backstory paints the straight one as a jock hero while
the gay one's mocked as a sissy. The brothers grew up in Connecticut. I was furious at this bald manipulation of my work,
the slur on my reputation, but my reaction was as nothing
compared to Tony's. He left a sobbing, guilt-racked message
on my machine: "I never wanted to hurt you, Paul. You were
just being my friend."

He simply couldn't understand how this woman could
have talked and joked with him and praised his grit, then
shifted gears and spewed this wretched travesty. At his own
peril he'd forgotten the Didion rule of engagement. My own
phone was already ringing double time. I savaged *Newsweek*'s
irresponsibility. It was just what abused kids feared the most,
that no one would believe them. Nancy Drew's text was riddled with AIDS-phobia. I told *The Wall Street Journal* that I'd
never met Philip Roth either, but it hadn't crossed my mind
that he didn't exist. I told *The Washington Post* that I couldn't
very well have written Tony's book, so busy was I writing
Vikram Seth's.

I told David that he had to convince the Johnsons to let a
reporter come and meet him. Reluctantly they assented, inviting Leslie Dreyfous from the Associated Press. She spent an

hour talking with Tony, assuring herself that this was the very kid she'd interviewed over the phone. AP prepared a story refuting *Newsweek*'s, detailing the visit to the Johnson home. By week's end other news organizations had distanced themselves from *Newsweek*. One of the magazine's editors remarked offhandedly to the *Post* that they no longer believed I had written the book, but that was the sum total of their retraction and apology.

I was advised by my lawyers not to say a word to *Newsweek* in my defense, but to wait and see if the libel would go so far as to merit a lawsuit against them. All parties assured me that the magazine was being inundated with outraged letters. *Newsweek* had so far made no direct attempt to contact me, but I had a call that week from David Ansen, an old friend who served as the magazine's film critic. Him I called back. He was clearly red-faced with embarrassment and swore he hadn't heard anything about this flap till now, because he'd just flown back from Cannes where he'd been covering the film festival.

"David," I declared in a withering tone, "you realize how nuts this whole thing is. Why the fuck would I want to write under a pseudonym? It's all I can do anymore to finish my *own* work."

Harrumphing sympathetically, not really wanting to get into it, David admitted he'd been asked to call by the editors, who hoped I would be willing to talk to one of their writers. It didn't have to be Nancy Drew herself.

"They've got to be kidding," I retorted. "You think I'm going to *dignify* this *National Enquirer* bullshit?"

Yes yes, he understood. He was more eager to get off the phone than I was.

We had to wait three weeks—till the June twenty-first issue—to hear the upshot, what turned out to be the second bowl of Eisenhower's snots. Indeed, *Newsweek* had printed several scathing letters. Amy Amabile, executive director of Northern Lights, an AIDS empowerment organization:

> *Your article is a perfect example of why there are laws to*
> *protect the confidentiality of minors and people with AIDS:*
> *many so-called journalists are willing to expose and exploit*
> *people with AIDS and victims of child abuse for the sake of*
> *a story.*

She went on to describe her own two-year friendship with the
young man, adding that Tony was serving now as editor of
the Northern Lights newsletter. The director of the Make-a-
Wish Foundation assured the magazine that they didn't just
arbitrarily grant wishes, that they didn't act without painstaking
documentation. Best of all was Tony's letter, a fierce declaration of his reality:

> *I exist; prove to me that you do! There is something unreal*
> *about a reporter who can joke and laugh with a person and*
> *then turn around and suggest that person does not exist.*

But *Newsweek* gave no quarter, upping the ante of its pit-
bull tactics, as if this story were as big as Watergate. They
pointedly dismissed the AP account of Leslie Dreyfous and her
visit to the Johnsons. "Paul Monette, who did not return calls
for *Newsweek*'s story, has since publicly and vehemently denied
Newsweek's suggestion that he might have written or helped
write Tony's book." The only call ever made to me was David
Ansen's, which I returned. But by now the little lies were
blown off the board by new heights of investigative gobbledygook:

> A spokesman for Manhattan District Attorney Robert
> Morgenthau said, "Our office has no institutional
> memory of this case." Officials in the New York City
> Police Department's Pedophile Squad and in the Spe-
> cial Victims Squad . . . could not recall a case resem-
> bling this one.

Quick, somebody go get Nancy Drew a Prozac! Of course there were no records in their files, because the whole story had taken place elsewhere. Place-names had been doctored to protect the victim, as the publisher made quite clear on the copyright page. It's standard procedure; I'd done the same thing in *Becoming a Man*. The magazine's update ended with a flourish worthy of *Dragnet:*

> Apart from Dreyfous, no individual has come forward
> to claim he or she has ever met Johnson in person.
> *Newsweek* continues to report the story.

How's that for playing hardball? So far as I know, their further investigations haven't posted a trenchcoated gumshoe outside my house. My phone remains untapped. Curiously, what Nancy Drew failed to investigate from the get-go was the parallel between her own debunking of Tony Johnson and the forty-year campaign to deny the truth of Anne Frank's *Diary*. In Europe there's a whole crypto-fascist industry whose only raging purpose is to prove that the *Diary* is a Zionist hoax. All part of a master plan to deny the Holocaust. Not crypto at all in fact, but put forth boldly by so-called scholars, and repeated often enough that in the end it becomes just another breeze in the climate of opinion.

I don't know why we expected any more of the media, those of us who nursed the publication of Tony Johnson's story. Not this summer anyway, infected as it is with shrieking bulletins about Heidi Fleiss (Madame to the Stars) and the Menendez killings and Michael Jackson's trial by headline ("At eleven, more celebrity reaction to the Michael Jackson story!"). Not to mention Woody and Mia. "Tabloid" doesn't mean anything anymore because there's nothing else.

But the *disappearing* of Tony Johnson's account of the unaccountable world is rather more sinister. Because it's a way of denying AIDS as well as him. And a hundred years hence, when all the tabloid victims of 1993 will be dust and ashes, the names no longer ringing the teensiest bell, the course of the plague will still attract the bewildered gaze of history. And when the Elvis sightings no longer fire the populace, and everyone has chewed Howard Hughes's two-foot fingernails to the quick, the storm troops of revisionism will trumpet their distortions from the rooftops.

So Nancy Drew, as it turns out, has just got an early start on the trivialization of AIDS. A picture from Cobb County, Georgia, in the current issue of *The Advocate* shows a crusty old coot proudly displaying a placard which reads PRAISE GOD FOR AIDS. If things get tame at *Newsweek,* I'm sure there's a good position available at the *Cobb Gazette,* or whatever they call their hate sheet down there.

One small piece of advice, Nancy: Don't forget to bring a lot of sugar. A boxcar full, because the snots get harder to swallow every day.

SLEEPING
UNDER A TREE

"I'LL SLEEP when I'm dead," declares my friend Dr. Barbara, petulant almost, as if she's far too busy running her clinic to waste good time in bed. Except in her case the lack of sleep is due to the throb of pain, for she is four years into the miasma of bone cancer, having exhausted all the "easy" treatments. Yet she refuses to languish now in a fog of Demerol, barely conscious of the fiery advance of autumn in the glade outside her window. And so—over the protests of her own doctors—she drops the milligram level, weaning her body from relief to get her mind back on course.

Not that she's ready to don a white coat again, or even to hold out hope of resuming her rounds. She possesses too keen a sense of reality for the bootstraps brand of magic thinking. The clinic has been passed on to her hand-picked staff of doctors, even though officially at least Barbara is merely on hiatus, a medical leave. That euphemism is a measure of their boundless esteem for her healing gifts—their hope for her return. The reality was clear enough two weeks ago, when she stepped out of bed and felt her ankle snap like a leafless twig.

Her patient-load of outcasts hasn't been given the least hint. To them, Barbara's a force of nature, something on the order of a household goddess, the world without her inconceivable. They pay her with guava jelly and the feet of chickens ritually sacrificed and bled, the latter an especially signal honor. Then they cook up the chickens for dinner, never quite long enough to kill the microbes, so the ones with AIDS end up with toxo. The taint of poverty always ends up in the viscera—bacterial, viral, fungal, all manner of rotten colonies. I suspect those so afflicted don't sleep much either, between the vomiting and the runs. But then they have no expectations otherwise, where life itself comes down to a chronic bad gut, nothing to be done about it unless they put it in Barbara's hands.

By contrast, I suffer a wimp's insomnia—no pain unless the itching counts, no place to have to get to in the morning. The ravages, in other words, are purely existential. If I weren't so prone to whining it would just be par for the course of things, hardly terminal in any case. Besides, I can't possibly sleep as little as I imagine, though the most minimal of morning appointments—leaving the car to be serviced, a two-minute blood draw, eleven A.M., the only available slot at neurology—will tend to find me rigid as if on a marble slab all the night before, waiting for the alarm to ring.

Forget about catching an early flight (in my case, anything before two in the afternoon). My psychic seat belt is fastened as soon as I get into bed, tossing and tumbling till I ball myself in a fetal crouch, the nearest I can approximate the crash position. And a single time zone change, or even daylight saving, a princess and a pea's worth, puts me out of synch for a week.

Insomnia is practically the original sin when it comes to crying wolf. Simian hominids in caves presumably complained of sleepless nights—a spur of rock in the den that jabbed them in the kidney, a mouthful of straw from their makeshift pillow. Even back then, nobody really gave the problem half an ear.

You didn't sleep last night—so sleep tonight. Or take a nap. What's the big deal?

Implicit in the sleeper's want of sympathy—those blessed folk who can turn themselves off like a light—is the suspicion that the sleep-bereft exaggerate. You didn't sleep *at all?* they ask with incredulity. And to be fair, we who are the exiles of the dark aren't above embroidering the long night's vigil. Perhaps the whistle was blown most forcefully on *that* technique by Proust himself, whose Tante Léonie would summon the household every morning in Combray, to bemoan her wide-eyed night of anxious wakefulness, counting the agonized hours as they chimed on the village clock. Only to forget herself five minutes later, soaking up her tea with a *madeleine* as she started in discoursing on her dreams, so vivid and so populous they've left her utterly limp.

Insomnia's midnight country is a sort of parallel universe, lunar and featureless, so it shouldn't come as a revelation that most people haven't been issued a visa. Or that they harbor a secret certainty that it's all our own fault—at best a failure of will, at worst a proof of guilt and shame, Poe-like in its intensity, blood seeping out of the walls. What the uninitiated can't seem to understand is the core banality of our empty nights. We may see ourselves in zombie terms, as a species of the undead, especially when we gaze at our gray and clammy faces and raccoon eyes in the mirror. But we most definitely lack the glamorous enervation of the vampire, pricked by insatiable hunger and a ravening of need, the fallen-angel mascot of the waking night.

Really, we are if anything the opposite of vampires. All we desire is sleep, the very thing that eludes us. In that half-moon state the carnal is about as appealing as an emetic. The loneliness may be unbearable, but the last thing you want is company. And when dawn finally streaks the sky with pewter and coral—damning proof of another lost night—then Dracula gets to fold his Batman cape, pull up his stone sarcophagus

lid like an eiderdown, and drowse away the indifferent daylight. Whereas we, the living, barely half-alive by morning,
have to rise from the twisted sheets and face the quotidian
world and keep our promises on coffee alone.

It was not ever thus. In my stunted adolescence, sleep was
the only reliable escape from the freakish burden of the body.
A virtual coma that extended twelve hours at a stretch, with
nary a complaint even from my bladder, nothing to interfere,
as if I traveled the dark with the constitution of a camel. This
was mostly weekend fare, of course, to make up for the rev-
eille call of the chapel bell at school, and dozing through "A
Mighty Fortress Is Our God," the spiritual equivalent of castor
oil and gelid porridge.

By the time I got to college one could get away with
sleeping in on a much more regular basis, dead to all eight A.M.
lectures (physics invariably) and strolling into The Nineteenth
Century Novel at eleven, balancing a double cup of java and
a powdered doughnut from George and Harry's. I think my
ancient lecture notes on Thackeray still bear a fine snow of
powdered sugar, as if the FBI had been dusting for prints.

Now it did not require an advanced degree to recognize
the linkage to depression in all of this, nor the hiding under
the covers that went hand in glove with the bleak condition
of sleeping alone. But if you're going to be despondent all
day long, you're probably better off unconscious. Interestingly,
insomnia is equally symptomatic of despair. Given the choice,
I'd take the coma any day.

But then when I started falling in love—or at least confusing it with sex—the spell of anesthesia lifted. I crawled out of
the cave of self like Rip Van Winkle, blinking at the light.
Suddenly I could stay up half the night, alternating embraces
with out-of-season plums, or running outside buck naked to
make angels in the snow—and *still* manage to make it to
school to teach my eight o'clock Senior English, with only the
barest post-coital yawn to betray me.

Is it just that being happy is better than sleep or anything else? Years on end, I don't recall a single night staring at the ceiling. Even when I would brazenly order an iced café au lait for last call at the Casablanca. Then I would put the night to work at writing poems, the self-appointed life of the solitary candle. No more sleep than Keats's nightingale, singing being as good as dreaming.

And when at last I found my way to Roger—eros and spirit and mind in perfect balance—the night was never solitary again. Within two years I'd given up my day job—those seniors agape with boredom over *Paradise Lost*—to take up the frontier challenge of writing freelance. Filling the day with paroxysms of typing, the evening saved for Roger always, but once he'd gone to bed a last flight of revisions and a sketch of the next day's plot. Sometimes it was two or three in the morning before I'd creep into bed beside him—but oh what safety was there then, what seamless merge of reverie. Falling into syncopation with his breathing, I was out before I knew it. Before I could even give proper thanks to whatever god of harmony had fated us with night after night in one another's arms.

The night didn't turn on me even when the writing started coming hard, four or five years later when I hit the skids of Hollywood. I'd lay down a patch of midnight dialogue, trying to keep it shallow for the overseers who couldn't swim. In a fit of dissatisfaction I'd get in the car and cruise the Boulevard, radio wailing the drunken sorrows of Country/ Western. Or stand at the back of a bar out of Dante, lost in the smoky shadows, nursing a beer like bitter herbs.

Pointedly unavailable. Until such time as I drew the attentions of those to whom unavailability was the very musk of turn-on. And then following one or another home to his digs in lower Hollywood, to have a go at Eros detached. The spoor of the trail nearly always more engaging than the act. Lastly, the flight from naming names, the merest swipe of a towel and

I'd be dressed and out the door. Fleeing those plaintive words that veteran nightfolk would sooner have their tongues cut out than utter: *Will I see you again?*

And even when it was three or four in the morning by the time I beat it home, I curled to sleep beside Roger the same as always, out like a light, sound as the bottom of the sea, untrammeled by guilt or hypocrisy. That would all come soon enough, in the train of the calamity. I come from a generation of queers who valued carnal freedom at all costs, to whom faithfulness was the rankest sort of bourgeois folly. Faithfulness to what? The riddled vows of heteros? Well, no— but then I never got the hang of sportsex either, the etiquette of meaning nothing, pleasure for its own sake. Not for want of trying, believe me. And while my back was turned, so to speak, the night recoiled on me with the kick of an M-16, shooting Sleep between the eyes and leaving me the carcass for a bedmate.

Like so much else that would never be the same again, it began the day of Roger's diagnosis—or more to the point, the night before. I was alone in our bed at home while Roger spent the first of a thousand and one nights at UCLA. Figuring over and over the odds of the next day's lung biopsy, already knowing in my heart that it wasn't a winnable match.

And once the doom had fallen—two weeks back and forth to Room 1028 at the Medical Center, Roger husbanding all his strength to recover—I began the twenty-four-hour day. A class-A insomniac will tell you there's no difference in the end between the dark and the daylight. You are just as witless, just as glazed, just as alien to any life you thought of as your own. Except by day you are actually falling into catnaps, no matter how inappropriate the setting. Slumped in the subway past your station, sprawled at your desk in a parody of cardiac arrest, as likely to pitch over into your plate as negotiate a forkful of food. And a holy terror behind the wheel.

Within days I was pleading for pharmaceuticals, who never

took a sleeping pill except on intercontinental flights, trying to cheat those time zones. I was so wired and frantic that I had no trouble getting scrip, whatever I wanted. A kid in a candy store of slumber. I started on Halcion by night and Xanax by day—but "only as needed," warned the doctors. Oh, reason not the need. These things only work for a while, of course—but offer in the short run a dreamless black hole to crawl into, midnight to dawn, succeeded by the tranquil float of a nerveless day. They worked for a matter of weeks, and then they backfired. This was well before the Halcion controversy, when the drug was fingered for various psychotic episodes, people confusing the local post office with the Vietcong or blowing away their bowling league.

But I kept the regimen up long after it made no difference, and probably would have been yelling in the checkout line at the Mayfair with or without the drugs. I remember thinking that a man could probably live for months without sleep, as long as there was someone beside him to protect. Roger after all was the one who required the restorative of a night unbroken: It was enough sometimes to listen to him breathe, one arm around him lightly as if to prove anew every second that he was still alive.

Six months later he lingered closer to death than life, the first of the experimental drugs having proven a better murderer than cure. I was delirious from keeping vigil; hadn't worked in months, but by then we were counting the days to AZT, the so-called miracle breakthrough that brought a whole generation of us to the brink of an early grave. But who knew then that science could get it all wrong; or that the drug conglomerates never met a disease they couldn't prolong the suffering of, if the price was right? All I know is, I had to set the alarm at four-hour intervals, day and night, and mix three IV bottles in a glass of juice and somehow feed it to Roger without really waking him up.

Here at least I swear that I'm not whining. This part had

nothing to do with insomnia proper. It was a privilege, frankly, to have so clear a purpose for keeping watch all night. I recall thinking the same as Barbara, *I'll sleep when I'm dead,* when what I was covering up was the truth I couldn't swallow: that I'd sleep when Roger was dead. The last six months of his blindness, the drenching sweats all night long, helping him change before he took a chill—it was all in the nature of having a night job, the graveyard shift in a factory that manufactured hope, or at least the illusion of endurance.

I took my forty winks when the nurse arrived at eight to set up the morning IV drip. And when one day she came in to shake me awake because something was very wrong, I bolted up as if I'd been caught sleeping at the wheel. Too late: the ship had already run aground. In the tortured final day and a half I watched Roger go from horrorstruck half-consciousness—fighting it like drowning just to take my hand, or later to moan my name when the brain shut down his power to speak—to full-bore coma, a body that couldn't do anything now, not even breathe on its own.

I'd been home in bed a couple of hours, a handful of pills barely keeping me under, when the phone call came at six A.M. to say it was over. And almost exactly four years later, September instead of October, I'd barely shut my eyes when the phone rang just after four, to say that Stephen was gone. Victor, who was holding me together at the time, took the call in the other bedroom, but I think I've never stopped hearing that twice-tolled ring in the night.

For the longest time now, probably since my own first incarceration at Midway Hospital (4 West, the plague unit), my sleepless nights have been marked by a weird anomaly. I read till three or four when the drugs kick in, heavy-lidded at last, and I douse the lights and drop off like a stone in a well. Only to come to, goggle-eyed, precisely an hour later, more often than not in a panic, still waiting for that call. Sometimes the ghost of an echo, as if I've already missed it. And that's when the real insomnia sets in, the hours that seethe with dread. You can almost hear the stonecutters chiseling your name.

It's questionable whether you needed quite such a detailed history of my sleep loss. (Not quite as bad as Stravinsky, at least, who regaled the breakfast table every morning with the minutest details of his bowel movements.) But because I've hit a new phase these days, unlike any that's gone before, I find myself following the thread backward over the course of the long night journey that's brought me here. The past as prologue.

You would've thought—*I* would've thought—that this startled waking to the ringless phone was a setup to force my brain to focus on my own dying. Unconsciously perhaps, but that's not how the scenario plays out; especially the bleak ennui. I stumble into the bathroom for a pee, batting away at the still unfocused dread like a cloud of flies about my head. Trying to stay thoughtless, no matter how rattled I feel. But even as I'm settling back in bed, the latest crazy topic of the night hooks its talons in me.

And I start dissecting the weather report, for example— not the weather, just the report. In Los Angeles the TV weathermen are a pack of whinnying ghouls, so perky and so upbeat they bring on a curl of bile before they even reach their time-lapse satellite maps. You realize they feel personally responsible for sunshine, as if they constitute the front line of the California good life. No matter if it's 103 out there in the valleys, a veil of smog the color of sherry, they act as if everyone else is as delirious as they are.

In other words, a perfect day for the beach—still frozen in time for them like Frankie and Annette, white kids riding the waves, tossing beach balls, cooking wieners, and never of course going further than first base. When in fact nobody but the urban underclass with nothing to lose would venture onto the beach at Venice or Santa Monica anymore, *West Side Story* in bikinis and jams. The bay itself slicked with the lime-green foam of industrial effluent, storm drains spewing medical waste and PCBs.

And when on occasion it rains they clearly take it hard, these guys, as if they've betrayed our very dreams. They mope over the swirl of clouds on the map, divining a break in the storm as if they could wish it away by positive-think alone. I don't know anyone anymore, natives especially, who doesn't welcome winter's changes, coastal fog and drizzle and torrents down the canyons. But nobody seems to have told the tele-vangelist pep boys, with their Palm Springs Florsheim tans and somewhere, doubtless, the first budding wart of melanoma.

Now what could this possibly matter, to make it worth an hour's tossing on a bed of nails? What prodigies of displace-ment must be at work? Sometimes I think I'm preparing a master list of what I will gladly leave behind when I'm out of here. But it isn't the weathermen really—it's that I can't be out in the heat of the day anymore myself, because I'll end up feverish and woozy. Meanwhile, the city of golden promise is falling to pieces as surely as my body is: Beirut meets Calcutta. And I am as powerless to stop the civic collapse as I am the corporeal one. You want the world to flourish even as you lose it, if only to give you a context worth the fight to stay above water. Or a certain altruism comes to wrap you like a lap robe, nudging you toward acceptance of your fate as you bequeath the rivers and mountains, the Rembrandts and the Beethoven string quartets, to generations yet unborn. The fu-ture of the spirit.

But it's not working out that way, because banality has flattened the earth like a series of monster typhoons, and the weathermen haven't even noticed, blind as they are from star-ing at the sun. Besides, the weather's the least of it. I turn on the radio in the car—forced to venture out in the heat because doctors don't have night hours—and the airwaves fairly

crackle with right-wing demagogues and shockmeisters, pur-
veying their white hate with a standup topspin. The old bullies
from the schoolyard, becoming Big Brother in front of your
eyes—or ears, in this case.

And the local TV anchorwork no better than the sunshine.
Huge segments given over to the separation of Siamese
twins—Baby Jennifer having to die to give Baby Melanie all
of the heart, with updates by the truckload till Melanie too,
alas, buys the ranch. In fact, there's always some kid languishing at City of Hope, waiting for a liver and kidney. Or
mauled by pit bulls (urban division) or a mountain lion (rural
division). Have I grown so callous that I've ceased to care
about these hapless tykes, or their little friends who peer from
every milk carton? No, I think it's the tone of forced sincerity
that gets me, the icky tug at the heartstrings, with footage of
weeping parents on the hospital steps, thanking us all for our
prayers.

Well, don't thank me. I'm too busy seeing through the
sentimental dreck to the millions of kids they wouldn't touch
with a ten-foot pole—the kids who are dead inside from daily
beatings, the ones incested by Mom and Dad, the starved and
the freezing, force-fed God as a sort of Mob enforcer. How it
rankles, the cheap-shot pretense of giving a shit about Little
Billy's kidney, exonerating them of all the damaged children
who would fill their segments twenty-four hours a day and
still not make a dent.

Again, what earthly use are such opinions from Paul Monette's *Overnight News*? Not a very popular attitude, recoiling
coldly from plucky Billy and Baby Melanie. But the surge of
insomniac madness doesn't care a whit for the niceties. It's
stuck like a bad witch who can't stop picking the scab off
every spell, rooting the pus ever deeper. It's Rumpelstiltskin
stamping in glee around his fire in the woods, waiting to
snatch a baby from its mother's arms. You don't even want to

know what goes through my head when a Christian school
bus full of campers misses a turn and lands belly-up in a ditch.

Feelings I wouldn't dream of entertaining by daylight, or
admit to anyway. Blowing off the rage, perhaps, after watching
everyone I loved die without a whisper of notice from anchor-
dom. Not to mention the Stepford Christians, who'd like to
burn us heathen at the stake. Note how they didn't proclaim
the Great Midwest Flood of '93 as a mark of God's wrath,
punishment for sin—or Hurricane Andrew in Florida; no
smugness about God having had a hand in that. No Christian
Supremacist suggesting that living on a flood plain or a lowland
swamp was after all a "lifestyle choice," so it served the whole
lot of them right to be wiped off the map.

In the dead center of the night I stoop to their level of
slime, heaving it back at them curse for curse—inoperable tumors and financial ruin, their children fallen into deep ravines
where no one will hear their cries. The morning-after hang-
over is enough to make me keep such things to myself, but
there's something dwindled in the soul from yielding to such
nastiness at all.

My own fault, surely, for channel-surfing the local news
from eleven to midnight, when *The New York Times* is tossed
on the front steps, Puck going down to retrieve it and drop-
ping it at my feet. So my head is fairly teeming with bad news
by one A.M., the up-to-the-minute stuff that assures fresh fester
for nightmares. The self-anointed saints of the New Age, with
their chipper dictum that AIDS can be fun, eschew the reading
of anything too real at any time, but especially last thing at
night. All well and good unless you were born with a congeni-
tal bad case of reality to begin with, indelible as your thumb-
print.

You may wonder why I don't just hang it up and go heat
a saucepan of milk and browse through something neutral,
Horticulture perhaps. In fact, I already do a glass of Ovaltine at
one A.M. and again at seven. The drug to keep my brain in

the ballgame requires dosage four times a day, to be taken with fats; and the doctors all concur that milk's not fat enough. I need to dump in a scoop or two of Haagen-Dazs, and a doughnut on the side wouldn't hurt. All of which tastes in the deeps of the night like the jar of old bacon grease my French grandmother used to keep on a shelf above the stove.

And you don't understand the addiction of insomnia if you think it responds to a walk out-of-doors to contemplate Orion and the Bear, or a dose of P. G. Wodehouse for merriment's sake. No, you stay in your bed in the dark and wait, forlornly of course, to snatch at sleep if it so much as hovers within your grasp. The only other action officially sanctioned and by the book is a check of the luminous dial on the bedside clock. But the rules are strict. You may check the time every couple of minutes, but you may not fixate on the sweep of the second hand lest it mesmerize you and get in the way of the night's agenda of cursing and minutiae. It goes without saying that you've long since rid yourself of any ·clock that ticks, as being certain to drive you right over the edge—Poe country again, the hammer of "The Tell-Tale Heart."

Keeping current with your enemies, of course, is standard thread in the warp and woof of nightwork. Not much to add when it comes to the latter-day Nazi All-Stars, Falwell and Robertson and Sheldon on first, second and third, the whole American Family Association cheering from the dugout, Gary Bauer as the nubile batboy. By way of National Anthem, they cover their hearts with their caps and sing "Tomorrow Belongs to Me" from *Cabaret*. You can run through that whole gang like rosary beads, at breakneck speed. They have long since been elevated to the Hall of Fame of bigotry—a Cooperstown of hate—so they don't require an insomniac waste of breath unless they've surfaced on the news that day with an especially loathsome slur. Hitting one out of the park, so to speak.

But there's always, always someone new to add to the roster. Arsenio's guest tonight is . . . President Clinton on sax! A rookie to be sure, but one who has attained to enemy status fast, after only a couple of times at bat. First there was his toadying to the Toad Queen of Congress, Senator Nunn of the indefatigable tongue—up the collective butt of the Joint Chiefs, his own mini–Tailhook Convention.

And yet that was mostly Presidential guilt by association. His own first foray into bigotry took place in the White House Rose Garden, in a colloquy with the People. Nudged by a Baptist preacher deeply troubled by the lifting of the military ban, Clinton frowned sympathetically. This Bill-who-will-promise-anything-to-anybody replied as to how the issue was all still up in the air, but that however the debate fell out, we mustn't be seen as *condoning a lifestyle.* The code phrase to end all code phrases, to us embattled queers the exact equivalent of shrinking from condoning *kikes* and *nips* and *woolly-heads.* The roses in the garden did not noticeably wither in shame, but then they are painted anew every night by a crew straight out of *Alice in Wonderland.*

And then there was his Neville Chamberlain imperson-ation on the tarmac in Denver, kissing the hem of Her Holi-ness himself, Uberstormführer John Paul II. In Denver, mind you, in rank defiance of *our* tribe's ban, Bitburg-in-the-Rockies.

But again, it's mostly guilt by association. Clinton waited till *after* his summer vacation to issue his own encyclical, *Religio Politico.* His first official appearance was at one of those Chris-tian prayer breakfasts—never been asked to one myself, but I gather they eat of the transubstantiated sausages of Christ. Any-way, Keynote Bill allowed as how the worst of our problems sprang from our having become too secular a society. There was far too much intolerance of the religious view of things, and especially of the practice of making political choices by way of the tenets of faith—voting the soul, as it were. Of course there was strict separation in the Constitution, a wall between Church and State, but surely (here a near seizure of ingratiation) there was room in the wall for a few doors.[1]

Not in *my* Constitution there wasn't any room, not for so much as a rathole. It takes a certain genius, I suppose, to get such an issue utterly backward—the most ominous development all over the world being the rise of religious fundamentalism, determined to eliminate all infidels and non-believers. The New Inquisition already upon us, mandating schools of cretinism for all good Christian children—where you unlearn the geology of the world but don't miss a day of praying for Little Billy's kidney and Baby Melanie's mortal soul. And the President's one of them, just another yahoo Baptist moron. Or so the sleepless night would have it. The bitter irony is that, given the chance to vote in '96 (don't hold your breath), I'd probably vote for him again. But then I'd vote for Donald Duck before allowing First Caddy Dan Quayle to occupy the Oval Office. Or waste a vote that might give any leverage to the Wal-Mart candidacy of Ross Perot, billionaire hayseed.

But heck, even we of the twenty-four-hour club have bought the conventional wisdom wherein *all politics is local.* Did anyone really suppose we were going to secure our rights by way of enlightenment from the top? That a good Bill Clinton would override the sodomy laws still extant in twenty-two states, or indeed take a stand on so much entrenched intolerance simply because it was the right thing to do? Not when tyranny is maintained—as it always has been—by the officers in the field and the prison guards with the cattle prods. Maintained by the likes of the Virginia judge who took custody away from a lesbian mother because her lifestyle was against state law. Rumpelstiltskin in black robes. Or the rabid used-car sales force that put over Proposition 2 in Colorado. We've

---

1. All of this was cribbed, I gather, from *The Culture of Disbelief* by Stephen L. Carter, New York: Basic Books, 1993. The Presidential book report.

come to understand that queers can't live in certain states anymore, the brownshirts growing in power every day. It's already
a new brand of civil war in the making, except the Confeder-
acy of Intolerance doesn't adhere this time to a North/South
axis. It's splintered everywhere, the smithereens in every up-
state village, every border town, the house on the corner of
every street—blinds drawn, no room in the garage for the car
anymore because of the weapons stacked there. Not a country
at all, really, but just a limping ad campaign for a past that
never was.

So what has all this to do with sleeping under a tree? Benign, undrugged, unvisited by nightmares. Free of curses. It's
a motif that seems to recur in culture after culture: the prince
in jeweled brocade in a Persian miniature, pillowed on a tuft
of moss beneath a cedar. Or a Hindu god, dozing on the banks
of the Ganges while a snow of cherry blossoms sifts about him.
Or a silver-wash figure on a Japanese screen shaded by bam-
boo, the seventeenth syllable in a haiku of dreams. For that is
what they always seem to be doing, whatever the local iconog-
raphy: dreaming the world.

Or as Roger once said, the week he died, when I woke
him from an all-day nap to take a doctor's call: "I'm sleeping
for everyone now."

Which was proof enough for the doctor that we were well
on our way to "serious brain involvement." Whereas I had
found the exchange piercingly wise and tender, and right on
the mark besides. Sleeping *le sommeil du juste*—the sleep of
the just—for all the rest of us, pursued day and night by our
compromises with nightmares.

It's the height of self-importance to see myself in the ob-
verse role, but I do sometimes. I think, *I'm having insomnia for
everyone now.* Making the best of a bad situation, because the
wise and tender thing seems so far beyond my reach.

So there you have a night in Paul's room. A one-way

harangue without benefit of context, railing at the sheer quotidian hairball of the day-to-day, the suffering of fools. Like an extended tour in solitary, positioned just under the drip of a Chinese water-torture. But not the whole night. Here I have to cop to the paradox of Tante Léonie, turning for a moment to the dreams that manage to track me down. Not the same as deep-sleep dreams, because these of mine inhabit the edges of an exhausted slumber, a morning jolt or two. Earplugs firmly in place and blackout curtains on the terrace doors, no ray of light to mock me for the new day I'm already missing.

They are more like seizures than dreams, actually, more immediate and jarring, with no narrative to speak of. Roger so close I could reach out and touch him, only he stares past my shoulder as if I'm not there. Or a panicky maze of rooms with too many doors, and though I don't know what I'm meant to do, I feel this desperate sense of unfairness that they don't seem to understand I have AIDS. I don't know who "they" are, but I have this burning urge to face them with my illness, being a sort of blanket excuse for why I can't keep up with them in the labyrinth.

Dreams of waiting—for doctors' appointments, for test results, for x-rays—all with the overriding feeling of suffocation from the mummy's tomb of an MRI. Sometimes just watching my mother, or Winston or Stevie, as they putter about the room. And they seem happy enough, or neutral enough, that I wonder if they've lost me yet. I am just the observer here, like Scrooge on the arm of Christmas Past. But it makes me feel such a pitch of melancholy that I can't go back and live there anymore. Not in the kitchen on Stratford Road, or the sunporch off it. Not in the Kings Road house as it was before the war. Not anywhere.

Dreams that seem to last split seconds, hardly the languorous undersea suspension that would allow me the scope to dream the world, as they do in the miniatures. And yet no less committed—in my mind, anyway—to finding the portal somehow into that oceanic ether, where I can project a future for my people. Dreams as wish fulfillment. But that isn't even possible without a more profound engagement with the night—which would also require me to give up the cursing and seething and political junk mail that keep me awake in the first place. I have a certain reluctance to part with the easy targets of my wrath, because they sustain me. But if I really mean it about the deeper dream of the world to come—my brothers' and sisters' legacy—then I know exactly what I have to do. To turn the tide of bile, I have to choose to hope.

A word that all but chokes in my throat. The practice of which is a rusty business, hardly even a memory now. As a commodity of the spirit, after all, hope has been most notable by its absence in the plague years—or at best discounted by so many false alarms of a medical breakthrough. Of course it's meant to be the posture of last resort, as in *All we can do is hope* and *Hope for the best* and, my personal favorite, *You have to have hope or you can't go on.* Well, no I don't. Not in an age that's up to its tits in blood, where genocide is anything but the casual outcome of aggression and stony indifference.

I've never really understood this business of Pandora. In the chronicles of myth she is sent by Zeus to the brother of Prometheus, who is far too wary to accept a gift from the gods. She brings with her as a kind of dowry a jar (not a box at all, a repackaging error of a later age) which holds a universe of evils and mortal pain thus far withheld from man. Fashioned out of clay herself, a Stepford wife if there ever was one, Pandora unscrews the lid of her jar because she is fated to. No moment of hesitation or any other feeling. And the evils escape like a flight of birds, a cloud of migration that dims the very sky. But as we were taught in the moral kindergarten of youth, Hope remained inside the jar, hiding under the lid, as a sort of consolation prize to the generations of humankind.

It is not reported what Hope was doing there, or whether

Pandora herself had exercised a human urge to compassion—
not unlike Prometheus himself, who stole a spark from heaven
to restore the gift of fire to man. Was it altruism that sought
to mitigate so much pain and suffering by the ministrations of
Hope, saving the best for last? And *whose* altruism, Pandora's
or the gods'? Personally I might've preferred her to hold Sleep
in the jar as a balm for man's estate. Perhaps I think that Hope
is as cruel as anything else she released to the four winds. Or
as Dr. Barbara put it in a recent letter, *the last horror let out of
Pandora's Box was hope.*

Nevertheless, even if all my fears prove true, I have to do
this thing. Have to hope. That the custody wars will go the
other way, reason winning out over bigotry, so that gay and
lesbian families aren't at risk of being scattered. (Because they
aren't going to stop saving children—not the ones they bring
out of failed straight marriages, nor the ones they adopt and
truly foster, nor the ones they conceive with a turkey baster,
that homeliest of fathers.) That the desperate queer adolescents
will survive the suicidal years and rise like the phoenix from
the ashes of self-hatred. That the closets will at last disgorge
their prisoners into the light. That we as a tribe will come
together to heal the earth with a passion equal to the death
squads of our fundamentalist foes. And that those who come
after never forget those of us who died of AIDS—who took
care of one another and, even when our strength had dwindled
to a fevered shadow, still fought the implacable agents of our
dispensability.

Not that I can impose that hope. I think my understanding
of the values they will need to keep them human in the face
of hate—keep them going—will coincide with theirs. But I
can't know for certain. Never perhaps have gay and lesbian
people been in such dynamic flux, mercurial in self-definition,
tuned to the ethics of survival. For all I know they will have
a guerrilla war on their hands, requiring stealth and night at-
tacks, the hiding of one another in attics.

So it will have to be a hope without any strings attached. Though I can't deny myself a certain utopian clairvoyance, imagining a time when gay and straight alike have reached a seamless self-respect, a love of those who are Other that goes way beyond accommodation. Making common cause for the sake of this brief and sinking island we call Earth. Sometimes, in a pitch of frustration over the inroads of our enemies, Winston will announce that we need a country of our own to be free in. Equal rights, of course, would do it, if our legislators would stop feathering their nests with the down of racists and Christian supremacists. And of course Winston knows there aren't any countries left—no secure frontiers—in a world that wallows in holy wars and ethnic bloodbaths.

No, we have to take our stand right here. There is no there. As someone who stopped saying the Pledge of Allegiance on the day they added "under God," who grew up with prayers in school that felt like the brainwash of Maoist thought control, I've come to appreciate the smallest gesture of resistance. Even as the Christian covens churn out diplomas to so-called psychologists committed to "reparative therapy" for queers.

Every act of resistance matters, every dream under the tree. Every Gideon Bible snatched from a hotel drawer and consigned to the nearest trash heap. Dreaming doesn't come easy to any of us queers, especially the young—who carry their closets and attics with them on their backs, as topheavy as Galapagos tortoises. And every single one of them, of course, has to find his own way to the dream country.

So, hope for the future wherever it takes us, allowing for all sea-changes on the way. We have only begun to understand how many of our gay and lesbian forebears perished in the fires of the Inquisition, a convenient Final Solution to the problem of the Other. And only begun to tap into the deepest well of our own reserves, the legacy of the shamans and the witches. (*Are you a good witch or a bad witch?*) No roles required, as long as we're free. And the gift of Sleep, a shady bower at every turn of Whitman's open road.

I've been there once or twice, though not in a long long time. But there's one moment that's stayed with me, when all the restorative forces conspired to align the sleeping and the dreaming. Roger and I were vacationing at the north end of Kauai, lazing in the limpid aquamarine of Hanalei Bay. By the third or fourth day we'd had a surfeit of sun—in truth, burnt to a cherry-red frazzle. Next morning we drove to the end of the road at Haena and started on foot up the cool and dewy trail that winds its way along the lower slopes of Na Pali, the vertical cliffs that face the northwest wind. No angle of repose between the jagged misty summits and the straight-down plunge to the battering surf. The definition of inaccessible and, with the drench of the trailside ferns, the moss and orchid overhangs, virtually the definition of green.

We did not know then that the trail had, for eons before the American Empire, been reserved for the feet of Hawaiian royalty. Since it's something like twelve miles from beginning to end, every step requiring mule-like purchase, it was doubtless the route of a vision-quest. And it ends in fact at an earthly paradise, the Kalalau Valley. No other way to reach it except this narrow trail, single-file—unless you approach it from inland, up Waimea Canyon. Which still leaves you at the summit, no way down into the valley unless you've developed wings.

No mystic baggage accompanied us as we threaded our way around ribbon streams that fell across the path with the force of cataracts. So many cascading runnels, it was like walking through a continuous downpour. It never stops raining on the heights of the dead volcano at the island's center—the wettest place on earth, they'll tell you. Still, we could see the sun on the water far below, a couple of hundred feet down from the trail. We met no one coming the other way, and there was no trail marker to reassure us. Along several stretches the trail was washed out, and we seemed to be scrambling across thin air, swinging by the roots of the upslope ferns, gorilla-fashion.

Then, somewhere into the third mile, you reach the sign you think you've been waiting for, staked into the earth, the inscription overgrown with moss. Reassuring it's not. It marks the limit of a tidal wave that bore down on Na Pali after an undersea eruption, drowning every creature in its path. Not much of a recommendation—depending on how you feel about lightning striking twice—for the patch of beach that beckoned from a shallow cove directly below. Though the disaster had happened a long time past—fifty years, as I re-call—the tremor in the heart remembered.

But we were nothing if not intrepid then. Since it was laughable to think we were going to make it all the way to Kalalau, traversing at such an inchmeal pace, we decided to take the escalator down to the beach. Like skiing without the skis, or the snow; swinging from root to root amidst an ava-lanche of mud. We emptied out onto the sand, no clue as to how we'd get up again, but meanwhile we had landed in an anteroom of Eden. Breakers throwing off clouds of foam as they thundered up the beach. The sun directly overhead, hot as magma. And back in the fold of the cliff face, a hollowed out half-dome in the rock, a cave of shade.

We went for a quick naked swim in the surf, paddling at the edges so as to keep clear of the undertow—whose sucking sound rasped like some leviathan breathing through a blow-hole, with an echo of whitest noise that filled the head like a Triton's horn. We sat cross-legged in the mouth of the cave and split our hiker's booty, a chocolate bar and two bananas. I remember wondering aloud if it was high tide or low, but we were already half asleep among the ferns, no energy left to contemplate a deluge from the sea.

Probably no more than a half hour's snooze, but depth was the issue here. Full fathom five and clear of all sea devils, till the pound of the surf around us had hushed to a whisper that echoed to our own breathing. Too deep for dreams, perhaps, like Wordsworth's thoughts that "lie too deep for tears." But just before I stirred awake I dreamed of Koolau—no more than a moment's embrace, but his face was unmarked and his limbs were whole. He didn't even have to tell me, for I could see that all was right again with him. The only thing I couldn't figure was how he seemed to know me.

We took our waking slowly, Roger and I, nothing much that needed saying as we came alive to a sanctuary that wasn't a dream after all. Later, when we had trekked back up to the trail and retraced our steps to the car at the end of the road, I told him about my meeting in the dream; wondering how I even knew it was Koolau, never having seen a picture of him. And not sure why it left me feeling so unaccountably happy. But then it's all a matter of degree, and those were the days when happiness seemed like a birthright.

Eventually I pieced together his story, more in the years that followed than I knew back then. Koolau the Leper, as he's called in every fragmentary reference, and in the title of a long-forgotten South Sea tale by Jack London. I assemble the evidence here by memory alone, doubtless having shaped it over the years into a folk tale of my own. But it happened; he was real. It must be a hundred years now, maybe more, but let's say twice as long ago as the tidal wave, a truer measuring stick for the boundaries of paradise.

It was a time when the bloodfire of leprosy was in full night bloom in the islands. Those who knew best—being the entrepreneurial forward line of American Interests—decided the hour had come for quarantine. And they began the systematic rounding up of the disfigured, transporting them to the "colony" on Molokai. But then that's what colonials do best, making colonies within colonies.

Yet when the troops arrived on Kauai and began to herd the infected, they encountered a proud resistance. Koolau was the lepers' spokesman. He swore they would never take him from the primeval home of his fathers. The troops fell back, outnumbered and nonplussed, cabling the Emperor in Washington himself. What to do? Within days it was decided the way it is always decided in the colonies: send the gunboats.

By which time Koolau had led his hobbled band, perhaps fifty strong, along the Na Pali trail all the way to Kalalau. The valley, a sort of oval crater that might have been the nest of the gibbous moon—a mile in breadth at the ocean end, three miles back to the sheer cliff walls—is completely defensible from any attack by land. Nothing more than a sentry force is required to guard the end of the royal trail where it enters the valley. The rim of the surrounding cliffs is too far up for an accurate shot, even if the people were visible below. Which they weren't, taking cover in the rain-forest shade and the natural caves in the mountain walls.

Even along the ocean flank, the valley ends in a line of cliffs, a steep descent to the tidal edge. So the gunboats couldn't land troops, because the lepers would have picked them off like ducks in a shooting gallery. The Navy blasted away, firing cannonballs that didn't quite make it past the valley's natural ramparts. A standoff, then, for several days. The lepers had water and breadfruit and taro in abundance, enough to last them forever. There are always bigger guns in the arsenals of Empire, but that would have meant bringing in ships from far away. If a real war erupted elsewhere, the Emperor might be caught with his pants down.

So the cannon stopped firing and a treaty was proposed by megaphone. If the lepers promised to stay and never come out, they could live in the valley unmolested—a leper colony by default. Agreed. Some say Koolau lived there thirty or forty years; an outpost of Eden and a tribe at peace. No one to make them pariahs anymore, and no one to recoil in horror from the breakdown of their bodies. A victory for dignity, it goes without saying, and maybe even a small payback for the wholesale rape of the islands, one of which had been sold to the entrepreneurs for a jug of rum.

I couldn't really say when the dream in the cave came to stand for me as a vision of hope, since it wasn't even a conscious quest. Three years later the sky turned black when the plague came down, and the blackness hasn't lifted by one candle flame since. The redneck preachers pelt our very funerals with rotten eggs, and we are just a hairsbreadth short of the escalation of hostilities to a shooting war. So far the cauldron of bigotry, with its Morning-in-America shock troops, has contented itself with bashing us to within an inch of our lives. The lynching comes next, and after that the extermination. I'm not going to be sleeping any better than I am right now— sentry unto Death, reading the moil of the night sky like a queer Cassandra, mad by definition.

So the memory of the dream encounter is that much more of a touchstone, blessed in slumber by the shining face of Koolau's act of resistance. You need only to have glimpsed it once to know there's a window out of all this black and sleepless night. Then you must use it to hope on. Key to the dream country where all your people are whole again, and the gunboats can't reach you, and the Empire of Hate is rubble. You and your secret dream of freedom are the tidal wave. Keep watch, every night if you have to. As for sleeping, you can sleep when you're dead.

MORTAL THINGS

MY LAST ENCOUNTER with feeling unworthy of worldly possessions—traveling light, as it were—took place on the occasion of my second Christmas, or perhaps it was my third. I toddled into the living room in my footed pajamas, my mother and dad waiting excitedly—Brownie box camera in hand, I suppose—to catch my glee at the sight of all those toys heaped under the tree. Apparently I walked right past the whole gleaming cache, made a bead for the end table by the sofa and grabbed a cheap glass ashtray, which I proudly clutched to my breast as I exited the toyshop.

I can't say I remember this. Or that the shifting tectonic plates of family history haven't ascribed the scene to my brother and various cousins instead. It's become a kind of all-purpose exemplar of a state of earthly innocence, a bare footfall behind The Little Drummer Boy in the family's psychic crèche. All I know is, we'd reached a whole different plateau by the time I was ten. Sharing a room with my brother under the eaves, I leapt from my sleepless bed at the first gray rose of dawn and beat it downstairs to check the Christmas haul.

Upon executing a speed read of the To/From tags, I raced back up to tell Bob, who couldn't get up himself till he'd put his braces on. Breathlessly I gave him the bulletin from the North Pole: "I got fifteen, you got thirteen." I'd like to think there wasn't a brag in that announcement, but of course there was. The one-upmanship of sibling life, factoring parental love to the decimal point.

Like Queenie the rat terrier in *A Christmas Memory,* fixated on the butcher's bone that Buddy hung high in the tree, "staring up in a trance of greed."

Not that I hadn't paid my dues in the court of bitter disappointment. Eating my share of that fat reality hoagie whose very bread and rancid butter insists that, as the Stones would have it, you can't always get what you want. I must've been about eight when we had a flier from the milkman, delivered at crack of day to the milkbox by the garage—two quarts every other morning, clear glass bottles with the cream at the top, sealed with a cardboard stopper. The announcement was collared around the bottle's neck: Glennie's Dairy was going to hold an auction the next summer, with prizes like skis and English bikes and season passes to Canobie Lake, the local amusement park.

But money would not be the currency. The bidding was rather to be done with those cardboard stoppers, so, *Kids, start saving them now!* It's a wonder I didn't succumb to lactic poisoning, given the gallons that I glugged down in the months that followed. My cardboard coin of the realm accumulated in a shopping bag behind the cellar door, augmented by donations from my Grandmother Lamb—who consumed one puny quart a week, but you took what you could get. On sub-zero mornings in the dead of winter the milk would sometimes freeze in the box, blowing its stopper with a geyser of white slush. The milk would then have to be dumped, but the stopper was still worth its weight in gold.

By summer I'm sure that shopping bag gave off a smell

like baby vomit, but I never did count my lucre till the week of the auction. Dad and I dumped it out on the kitchen table, tallying up 155 (157 counting the two in the fridge). The auction was set for Friday evening at the dairy. You have to understand that Glennie's was a purely local operation. (No match for Hood's, with its statewide distribution and regular mooing ads that sponsored the weather report on Channel 4.) Glennie's was the place we went for grade-school field trips, cheery and twee as Old Macdonald's farm, despite its row of tin-sided barns filled with cows attached to the automated milker, untouched by human hands.

It was a sultry August evening, slow to give up the daylight. We arrived and were herded to park in a fresh-cut field, and I tried not to feel deflated by the sight of those acres of cars. We made our inching way with the crowd through the pasture gate, gathering toward the wide circle of onlookers surrounding the makeshift auction stage, lit by strings of Christmas lights. Presumably the booty was piled behind the stage, but I had to take that on faith, given the fact that I couldn't see a thing over the wall of grownups who'd arrived there early. Too big to be hoisted on my father's shoulders, I had to hear second-hand what item was on the block. The auctioneer, used to selling pork bellies and the detritus of bankrupt farms, was talking so fast that I could hardly follow.

The first lot cried was a picnic basket, with a fine fitted interior, plates and linen and cutlery included, as well as a nest of Tupperware. Nothing that I particularly coveted. And I thought I must've heard him wrong when he bawled, "Who'll start the bidding at five hundred?"

I cannot convey the crushing weight of the next thirty seconds, hearing the bidding rocketing up to two thousand, three, then four. Only now, as my eyes adjusted to the dusk, did I see the resources we were up against. Trash barrels full of stoppers, burlap sacks and cardboard cartons that once held washers and dryers. The items that followed were all a blur—

a doll that wet her diapers, *going going gone* for four hundred. A deluxe Erector Set, complete with wrenches—*eight hundred once, eight hundred twice, sold to the man in the Red Sox cap.* Who as it turned out was our milkman.

There was no point in prolonging the agony, waiting for the three-speed Raleigh and the jungle gym. My dad shrugged it all off with a rueful laugh, and I did my best not to cry, though the lump in my throat was the size of a golf ball. As we threaded our way out of the crowd, I couldn't hear what treasure was next, but I hollered as loud as I could, "A hundred and fifty-seven!"

Various adults around us chuckled in sympathy, holding bags that looked even less commodious than ours. As we passed a rural fellow and his brood of squalling kids—a tableau right out of the dustbowl, worthy of Dorothea Lange—it was the father himself who looked to be holding back tears. Defeated by too much hope, a man who must've learned long ago that there was no free lunch. He caught my father's eye, and they exchanged a moue of frustration. Next I heard my father ask, "How many *you* got?"

" 'Bout three hundred," came the reply, but then he had twice as many kids as we did, who probably drank their milk by the pailful.

"Here, take ours," Dad declared, lifting the shopping bag out of my arms and handing it over. Just like that. And six months of hoarding stoppers—my sweepstakes project that came to nothing at last—vanished like the flush of youth.

I think I was angry with Dad at the time, giving the store away without even asking me, but that was sheer displacement. By the time we'd driven home in the wood-sided '49 station wagon, I understood what a practical gesture he'd made—not to mention generous. I recall he even apologized for the whole mess, as if he ought to have warned me all along that the best-laid plans fuck up. Then he bucked us both with a stop in Boxford for a Benson's ice cream cone. Dairy was clearly the leitmotif of the evening, if not of my entire eighth year on the planet.

And how have I done since then? Depends. But I've never forgotten that 157: when I came up short of the grades at Yale to make Phi Beta Kappa; whenever I've had to settle for a niggling book advance; especially when my T-cells fell that far, only off by a point or two. There was a time when I wanted it written below the name and dates on my gravestone: 157. Let the deconstructionists figure *that* one out.

And doesn't the lesson of that muggy August night still have its hooks in me? I've never bought a lottery ticket, even when the pot was soaring into the nine figures. When Winston and I were bound from Denver, passing the night in Vegas before the last push to L.A., I was constitutionally incapable of feeding the nickel slots. (Till he forced a roll of quarters on me and gave me my first lesson in the one-armed bandit—a lesson that never quite took.) Nothing is free. Bad luck being more to the point than good, why tempt fate by winning? Doubtless an old Puritan gene that taught me that even if I hit the jackpot—up to my knees in quarters, so to speak—I was likely to exit the Desert Inn right into the path of a bus or a drunken Eldorado.

Besides, it's the atavism of the crowd at Glennie's Dairy that's stuck with me—oh, including my own—the craning hungry faces of the townsfolk, just this side of a riot if they should come up empty-handed. A naked trance of greed indeed; not so very different from the players in Shirley Jackson's story, bound by a yearly madness that served to propitiate their darkest gods, only with stones instead of milk stoppers. "The Lottery" played for keeps, where blood kin snuff blood kin.

In my bookish adolescence I was a terrible snob when it came to things—imagining that the stuff of the mind was on a whole different level from the world of convertibles and power boats, snowmobiles and all the rest of that suburban loot which counted for glittering prizes. I read like a speedboat

myself, never pausing to catch my breath between *The End* of
one and the start of the next. I wasn't especially discriminating,
needing to fill up the empty hours when I wasn't pining for
boys to rut with. Reading as monkish distraction.

The hoarding came a bit later, giving up the library stacks
in the face of the burgeoning paperback boom. (Half the
queers I've ever met seem to have gotten it on in the stacks of
their youth, or at least in the downstairs loo. Another string of
missed chances in *my* book, too busy reading, holding my water till I got home.) I would even read while walking back and
forth from town, not so much as looking both ways at the
corners—thus the attendent screech of brakes that followed in
my wake. But once I started buying paperbacks myself, I became a virtual Evelyn Wood in my absent-minded wanderings,
possessed by the need to add yet another title to my bedroom
shelves.

By the dozen and then by the hundredfold—watching the
literary rows fill up as if my mind itself had found a physical
form, and gratifyingly solid in a way that milk stoppers could
never be. Reading for bulk, not content, like a power lifter
mainlining steroids. The whole process abated in college, stuck
as I was with groaning texts that took months to get through,
and no real desire to add their doorstop heft to my personal
collection. Besides, college was such a constant torment of romantic longing, pining worse than ever for those unattainable
boys who looked right through me. The one extended time
in my life when reading didn't matter—indeed, when I could
scarcely see the blur of words for all my hormonal madness.

Not till I was rudely thrust into the real world after graduation did I resume my bookish accumulation. Presumably
more discriminating, but ever more hyper to build a wall of
intellectual bricks, the book-lined study of my particular closet.
Haunting second-hand stores and bargain bins, and for the first
time acquiring volume after volume that I would never find
the leisure to read. Tomes that piled up on my desk and

bedside table gathering dust, till the sheer Malthusian geometrics of it all forced me to shelve them unread. What am I doing otherwise with the Holroyd two-volume bio of Lytton Strachey, a figure of not even marginal interest to me? Or the Belknap Press set of the Brownings' letters, florid and not my style? But then Anthony Powell's title has it exactly right: *Books Do Furnish a Room.*

I remember Roger beside me as I plumped the sixth volume of Mrs. Woolf's letters on the counter at Book Soup; and not so many years later Volume Five of her diaries. On both occasions Roger murmured, slyly but not judgmental, "Do you think you'll ever read it?"

The truth? No way. But by then the mere act of acquisition had taken on a life of its own—still trying to make up for the too-small book allowance left over from my prep school paycheck, not to mention an end run around that 157. These were more for reference than for reading, I told Roger, and more than that for providing a bracing view from my desk in the study. A harmless enough diversion, in any case, and hardly unique. Just being in a smart bookstore, redolent with the heady smell of print, a Dionysian pleasure going all the way back to Gutenberg. We all end up with too many books we wish we could absorb by a sort of osmosis, mind over matter.

In my case there was also the mind's sub-basement where I did my screen work, with its INTs and EXTs and arbitrary divisions into Acts—as far from theater's organic use of breaks as from the Acts of the Apostles. I would find myself staring idly at my wall of books across the room, my security blanket and shield, proof that my brain wasn't slowly leaking out my ears. And round about '83 deciding that brain death was imminent, I put myself on a schoolmarm's regimen of self-improvement, making up for all the lacunae of my so-called education. From *Robinson Crusoe* to *Lady Chatterley*, from *The Way of the World* to *Heartbreak House*, a delicious couple of hours late every night to no purpose but my own.

Then Roger got sick. From that moment I ceased to con-
centrate except on him, leaving *The Golden Bough* dog-eared at
page 221, as abrupt as the unfinished symphony of Schubert—

To this day the Sultan of Wadai must have no obvious
bodily defect, and a king of Angoy cannot be crowned
if he has a single blemish, such as a broken or filed
tooth or the scar of an old wound.[1]

And never to be resumed, ending the era of self-improvement for good. It's true that Roger and I passed the summer
before his death reading Plato aloud, or I did anyway, since he
couldn't see. And yet from the sudden onset of his blindness I
started jettisoning our books, like pulling out the stitches of
some vast needlepoint tapestry— *The Lady and the Unicorn,* say,
at the Cluny Abbey in Paris.

At first I put them in boxes, thinking I'd give them away.
But no library wanted them, too expensive to catalogue and
store, no matter how intellectually superior. The best I could do
was offer them to jumble sales at churches, fodder for the bin-
combers—twenty-five cents apiece as is, then finally reduced to
a dime on the final day of the fair. I began to play a ruthless game
of triage, especially when it came to Roger's cheap-bound classics from the French, so yellow and brittle with age that the pages
crumbled to dust in the hand. None of that sweet perfume of ink
and paper, but musty and final as ashes, like papyrus debris in the
ruins of the Library at Alexandria.

And when he died, I only accelerated the process. All slim
volumes of poems by the defiantly obscure. Any old textbook,
kept against the day I might teach again. There was room for six
hundred books on the shelves in the study and the living room

---

1. James G. Frazer, *The Golden Bough* (New York: Avenel Books, 1981), page
221. Citation from Plutarch's *Agesilaus.*

alcove. But we were way over our limit, books piled teeteringly on top of the once alphabetical rows, a veritable chaos of books bulging from every cranny. I determined to throw one away for anything new that arrived. Not that I was buying much anymore, but the books came in from the publishers—galleys bound and pleading for endorsement, every book on dying of AIDS and just as many about beating it.

Not that I didn't blurb my friends from time to time, especially the gay and lesbian ones, or rejoice at the fruits of their hard-won success. Rita Mae Brown remarks in her impish writer's manual that John Milton didn't go blind from any organic cause, but rather from reading unsolicited manuscripts. When I gave it up, it was partly that, and partly that I didn't respond anymore to the reach of other writers' imaginative cosmos. Nothing new to learn, not even that goosing twinge of envy that used to propel me through better books than mine. Whatever I needed to get through the night just wasn't available between book covers.

Late in his life Edmund Wilson used to send a postcard by way of reply to various inquiries. It went something like this:

> *Edmund Wilson does not*
> *( ) read unsolicited material*
> *( ) give after-dinner speeches*
> *( ) answer personal letters*
> *( ) write introductions*
> *( ) accept honorary degrees*

He'd check the appropriate sentiment and be done with it. The sour grump of which notwithstanding, I understand he had no time for anything but his own work, and was usually reading his way through Balzac, Turgenev, the Dead Sea Scrolls, or the whole of Canadian literature. A man who couldn't bear the quotidian.

It wasn't that I had such high-toned literary tasks as Wilson's, requiring all my time. Honestly, it was as simple as no longer opening books with a sense of anticipation, even wonder. I didn't want to read anything over again—not even Forster, the angel on my writer's shoulder. Or Iris Murdoch or Graham Greene or Flannery O'Connor, writers I'd read straight through, especially in those years when I preferred the feelings of fictive characters to life. Not even my own work spoke to me. No false modesty there, since nothing has stopped the near-erotic trailing of my finger along the spines of *my* shelf. But not to read.

Eternal regret: Forster was in residence at Kings College, Cambridge, in the summer of '66 when I was there. I passed his windows and thought about sending a note, but was far too shy to follow through. A music scholar I met last year told me I should've come by for tea to Forster's rooms, no invitation required, for he always delighted in new faces. A jolly time of wit and chortling laughter—the biographies never seemed to get it right about his irony—as long as you didn't overpraise his work. J. R. Ackerley, the *other* queer English writer in the generation after Oscar Wilde, was often in attendance. And if some new face went into gush mode over *Passage to India,* Forster was quick to parry, "Oh, but Joe has a book about India too. You must read that."[2] Now *there* was a mortal occasion not to miss, better than reading any day.

Oh, of course I've kept a certain quantity of literary totems I'd never part with—anything from the ancient world, but then that stuff's practically immortal. The fragments of Pindar and Sappho, the bawdy and vivid lyrics of Catullus and the knife-edge quips of Martial. And despite my scatterbrained excuse to Roger back in the days of Mrs. Woolf—*more for reference than for reading*—that's what I do with most of the books

---

2. J. R. Ackerley, *Hindoo Holiday: An Indian Journal,* New York: Penguin, 1984.

that remain. Following up on a line or two of poetry that I never quite committed to memory—or worse, had tried to improve on. Tracking down the moment in Jane Austen when Emma finally gets it through her head about Mr. Knightly. "If I loved you less," he tells her in the garden, "I might be able to talk about it more."

But even reading Sophocles, I start maundering in my head that I can't experience it in the original. Oh well, no time to learn Greek now. Garry Wills tells a lovely story about being arrested at a demonstration and having in his pocket a Greek New Testament. He remarks to a fellow detainee— libertarian anarchist Karl Hess—that if he had to know just one language besides his own it would be Greek, because its literature was suffused with the language of all the founding genres of Western culture. I can picture him reading the letters of Paul in the holding pen.

Then several weeks later Wills was hauled in again from *another* demonstration, and Karl Hess struggled through the crowd to his side. "Let's try to get in the same cell," said Hess, "because I've been working on my Greek verbs."

That is the sort of intangible I envy, not a matter of things *per se,* though of course requiring a text and a dictionary. Edmund Wilson experienced a frustration not unlike my own in his final decade—he who could read a dozen tongues, but couldn't master the nuances of Mandarin Chinese and Hebrew, not enough to claim them as his.

Intangibles, which books are not, though the contents are. Both in the collecting and dismantling of my library, I've surely been too caught up in the "thingness" of books, when what has really fashioned me is the sum of a thousand narratives and stanzas, the revelations of a writer's voice. Can't take any of that to the grave with me either, but probably up to the very brink I will die with a quote on my lips. A whisper of profundity that, if I have the breath left, I will doubtless supply with a proper footnote.

As for the act of writing itself, the tools of the trade have changed utterly in my lifetime. In grammar school I went through six years of the Rinehart method of penmanship, copying out pages of individual letters till we were deemed ready to essay a full sentence. In third grade we graduated from pencils to inkwells. Individual wells in the right-hand corner of each child's desk, and a black wood pen like a mini-conductor's baton, with a changeable nib at one end.

Learning the body English of dipping and then transferring ink to paper demanded rock-hard concentration. Woe to the kid who blurred his letters by applying too much ink. Of course we also had squares of blotting paper, but they were meant to be used sparingly, for words that didn't dry fast enough. We weren't, after all, in the business of making Rorschachs. Miss Alice Stack in the fourth grade, who came round every Friday with her thin-lipped watering can of ink to give us refills, actually made it a practice to check our blotters, factoring an excess of blot into our penmanship grade at report card time.

I still prefer today to write in longhand, though thankfully in the blotless age of the ballpoint and the Flair. In '83 I managed to make the transition to word processor (hateful phrase, like verbal Velveeta), kicking and screaming the whole way. My pre-Columbian computer is a vintage IBM, whose upgrading and updating I've avoided from the first, dashing the hopes of salesmen who long to bring me up to snuff. "But it's so *slow*," they tell me. "You could be into your file in two seconds." But I rather like the chugging and throat-clearing of the IBM, like an engine turning over on a frosty morning. And anyway, I don't want to go fast.

Thus have I eschewed both fax machine and laptop, even as they proliferate all around me. Absolutely everyone who knew I was at sea for several weeks last summer, hearing that I'd managed to finish two of these essays shipboard, remarked in chorus: "What did you use, a laptop?"

"No," I replied, "a pen." And in the face of their various states of shock, I added helpfully, "You know. By hand."

Hardly a day goes by that someone doesn't propose to send me something in a flash: "Here, I'll just fax it to you." After informing them that I haven't bought into that technology as yet (but ·as if its arrival is imminent; not wanting to imply that my house is lit by whale-oil lamps), I wait out the loss of words of my up-to-the-minute callers. "You could send it overnight mail," I suggest, in case they think their only other option is Pony Express. "All right," they reply, conceding defeat, but clearly aghast that they might have to wait in line at the local P.O.

So I am something of a throwback, no doubt about it. But I've also come to feel it as an acute pain in the region of the heart that writing by hand will be the hardest thing to surrender at the end. A few years ago in the British Museum, I remember poring over the "fair copy" of *Jane Eyre,* the final presentation draft submitted to the publisher. The hand was clear and unvarying, not a word crossed out or misspelled—a sure A+ in Miss Alice Stack's gradebook. And this was the standard back then: the patient copying out of near three hundred pages, with a rhythm of such repose that you couldn't fail to see what a physical act of pleasure it was, making that fair copy.

Or consider Francis Parkman, brilliant historian of the French and Indian Wars, whose own ill-health plummeted even further after his exploration and site research for *The Oregon Trail.* So debilitated was he after 1850, suffering from

> a complete exhaustion and derangement of his nervous system, a mental condition prohibiting concentration, and an extreme weakness of the eyes,[3]

---

3. James D. Hart, *The Oxford Companion to American Literature* (New York: Oxford University Press, 1969), page 634.

that he could often compose no more than six lines a day. Eventually he employed a metal grill that he would lay down over his manuscript as a sort of template, writing between the thin metal bars. Virtually blind for decades, he nevertheless produced some nine volumes of history, most of it still peerless a hundred years later.

But then patience was once the order of the day, and the physical act of writing was close to the operational definition of being a writer at all. Jane Austen wrote at a tiny desk in the parlor, and whenever someone entered the room she would swiftly slip the manuscript under the blotter or in the drawer. Not shy, not threatened, but ever alert to her social duties and somehow thriving on interruption, since the bustle and gossip and coming-and-going were her great subject after all. I assume it took her no more than a couple of seconds to pick up where she left off—quick as any modern software.

In the moving premonitory memoir of his approaching death from cancer, poet Donald Hall discovers that what he will miss the most are the dailiest of things. Padding out onto his porch to retrieve the morning's *Globe;* a quiet cup of coffee as he peruses the headlines; the dozen small nesting motions that bring him at last to his desk. Finally the picking up of his pen to start afresh. The things of life are so ordinary, the habits so engrained, that it's stupefying to think of them taken away. One wonders that the universe would bother to kill off such a modestly focused life, circumscribed by hours of quiet on every side.

Anyway, that's how I feel about having pen in hand, gliding along line by line on the trail of something new, usually something I haven't even dreamed of till it's written down. Such a small business—tactile before all else, a sleight-of-hand producing a squiggling Steinberg line that flows and flows— and the best proof available that I'm still breathing.

So even if books are not what they used to be, writing is. Of course the accumulation of pages has its own force of ego, bringing a thing to life; but every single stroke of ink feels shamelessly satisfying. Incremental, like the stitches of another sort of tapestry. Such that even if there seems to be nothing more to say—no lady, no unicorn, no ground of a thousand flowers—the needlework just won't quit.

A master woodworker I knew in Boston once told me that when he reached forty he found himself watching his hands all the time, alert to the merest slip of the saw that would leave him half a digit short. Till then, he said, he'd taken his hands entirely for granted, too many close calls at the jigsaw, so careless of the danger that he ought to be fingerless by now. That's how I think about going blind, something I'd not even considered till Roger's eyes were taken. And knowing that only a single medicine stands between me and sightlessness—a daily hour of IV drip, like a warmup to limber my neural muscles—I realize how killing it would be to have to give up my pen for a keyboard.

I still remember Roger signing his will a month before he died—a caricature of his gentle hand, by memory alone, and wide of the line he was meant to sign till the lawyer and I guided his pen to the proper spot. Blind isn't dead, I know that, but blind is no longer writing by hand, thus not writing at all. The pen can't live without the eye, nor the eye without the pen—not in my cosmos anyway.

I haven't addressed thus far, have avoided even, the big-ticket items of ownership—houses and jewels and paintings, miles of private beach. The possessions that go with power, so mighty and so various, but that finally lie in waste and adrift with sand, like the kingdom of Ozymandias. In my twenties I was possessed by a wanton envy of the rich and their lives of seemingly limitless possibility. I took no notice of the cautions of *Gatsby*—neither the hollow shell of the hero as he gazed across the water at the green light on Daisy's dock, nor indeed the uncontrollable tears of Daisy herself, burying her face in the soft profusion of Gatsby's shirts. Virtually every book about the moneyed that drew me in—from *The House of Mirth* to *Between the Acts*—was a cautionary tale. The stiff repressive social order; Marley's ghost dragging his strongbox behind him like ball and chain; story after story in which the possessor stood possessed, weighted with things, waiting for the glittering world of privilege to hit the iceberg.

None of it really deterred me, though, from wanting to get in the door. But the old Brahmin rich of New England— their faded drapes, moth-eaten cardigans, chipped old dishes their ancestor captains had hauled from China for ballast, tins of Welsh rarebit from S. S. Pierce—weren't quite what I wanted. No reckless glamour, no Bugatti with sable lap robes, no Baccarat flutes flung from the Murphys' terrace into the sea off Juan-les-Pins. I wanted to witness Croesus-rich, robber-baron rich, fuck-you rich. Enough of these latter-day Puritan rich of Boston, born with silver spoon in mouth and sucking it ever after like a lolly.

I had no idea what I really expected from such baronial encounters—sudden adoption perhaps, because I would prove such a perfect fit on the strength of wit and charm alone, the very frog they were looking for to elevate to prince. And when I finally stumbled on the very thing, it was by the sheerest inadvertence. A fellow English drudge at Sutton Hill School, seemingly churchmouse-poor as I, was bundling his wife and children off to Bermuda for spring break. They'd be staying with his grandmother, in a cottage behind the main house, a bare stone's throw through the sea pines to the beach. There were plenty of extra beds—would I like to come? I think it was the "main house" part that hooked me. I accepted before he'd finished inviting me.

And it was surely the grandest place I'd ever gained entry to, even if the "main house" proved something less than a mansion. A very old house with a white-limed ziggurat roof for catching rainwater, typical of the island style where fresh water was like gold. Shipshape—literally so—since most of the timbers and cedar paneling had been salvaged from ships that foundered off the point. A captain's desk and a couple of leather-strapped sea chests, fit for *Treasure Island,* and a bronze ship's bell on the front verandah to summon us in for meals.

Not big, as I say, but grand. With terraces opening out on every side, ancient coral paving pocked with lichen and moss, shaded by loblolly pines and bowers of jasmine. To the south a panorama of the lordly Atlantic, studded with coral outcrops that had brought all those ships to their knees in the old days. To the north and east the view to Harrington Sound, placid as a salt lake because protected from the open sea. But more remarkable still was the acreage of open land all around, so the estate was as rustic as it was private. One field was planted in Easter lilies, and another served as grazing land for half a dozen cows, who lowed as if they'd died and gone to heaven.

The "cottage" where I bunked with my friends was an old white-brick salt mill, cut from a coral quarry, fitted out now for guests and pungent with the sea—as if the walls still leached out salt, the concentrated perfume of a mid-ocean breeze. The days were casual to the point of near-delirium, swimming and walking the empty beaches surrounding the estate, exploring the caves the tide had gutted out of the coral. Three or four times we had lunch at the dock on the Sound, all of us diving like pearl fishers to bring up buckets of Harrington clams. Then each of us was given a razor-sharp clam knife and half a lemon. We sliced open the clams, revealing the meat still alive and quivering. A squeeze of lemon and we scooped them out and popped them into our mouths. Writhing against our tongues as we chewed them alive. It definitely took some getting used to.

So this was how the other half percent lived, with customs so rarefied I'd never even heard of them. And then there were the permanent residents of Grandmother's principality. Herself like the prow of a ship with a bun of snow white hair. Not a bit arch, though, or radiating anything like the superior air of noblesse oblige, scion though she was of near three centuries of island lineage, ancestors planted in the windblown graveyard out in Saint George's parish. A striking beauty still, though she must have been a knockout once, the most eligible of the princess class.

A quality she had apparently passed on intact to her daughter Margo, an Ondine sprite who must've been thirty that spring when I met her. Not a sprite anymore, of course, except in the portrait over the mantel in the library—but still with an orchid rarity about her even as she passed into full womanhood. With the angles and fluid grace and incandescent smile of Audrey Hepburn, born to wear designer clothes. Living that year with Grandmother, recovering from a messy divorce, with a pair of Etonian sons in short pants, Charles and Richard, whose company manners were rather too impeccable. Megs, as the family called her, always seemed to be gently teasing them to loosen up. But as they spent eight months of the year within the borders of their father's domain, looseness wasn't in the cards.

A Croesus in the flesh, this man, heir to a railroad fortune and platinum mines and tracts of timberland as vast as your average banana republic. Fell head over heels for Megs in the midst of a yachting regatta, and within two weeks had married her. The biggest blowout wedding in island memory, three hundred guests arriving by horse and carriage, all-night dancing at the Mid-Ocean Club, and a breakfast of pheasant at dawn.

Then he spirited Megs away from her luminous isle to the moveable feast of an entrepreneurial barony. Duplex on Fifth Avenue, an Adirondack lodge, the Middleburg Hunt in season, and a Moorish palazzo in Palm Beach. Trappings within trappings within trappings. I never heard it from Megs herself— the ennui of too many houses, the gathering panic of exile— but the family let you know. Delicate since Richard's birth; shouldn't have gone through it twice. A frailty that sapped her even now that she'd come home, and veiled references to surgery that mightn't have got it all—and me too stupid with dazzle to figure out that they meant cancer.

Still, she never spoke ill of Croesus—everyone else did—civil perhaps for the sake of the boys. But then, the boys had also sealed her claim to mythic stature, a *sotto voce* awe that trailed her like the whispers of the Furies. When Charles was born nine years before, he was officially Charles V, inheritor of the whole gilded century past—as if the railroads and the platinum were genetic. And when Megs came out of the anesthesia—a butchered delivery, it was said, calling to mind those clam knives—Croesus appeared before her in a burst of dynastic pride, presenting to Megs a tooled leather box, black velvet inside.

Containing a necklace of knuckle-sized emeralds, the very same that Napoleon had presented to the Empress Josephine. Josephine being Megs's middle name, and her husband a full-fledged emperor of commerce.

The night my friend from Sutton Hill told that story, vodka-and-tonic on the ocean terrace, his own wife piped up with the punchline: "When Richard was born, he gave her the rubies." The Empress's rubies, that is—a rope of blood-red stars from Burma.

In the speechless hush that followed, all I could think to ask was, "Did she get to keep them?"

"You mean in the divorce?" queried the teacher's wife. "Of course. But so what? They're just in a bank vault somewhere."

And that was that, the cautionary tale in a nutshell. You didn't even get to have the things you had. For wearing in palaces only.

"I don't know why she's still so sad," the wife went on. "He was a total prick to her otherwise, and she never cared for jewelry anyway." You felt the teacher's wife would have loved the chance to care for some herself.

Sad? Was that what she was? Not around me at least. We'd

hit it off instantly, the two of us, because I made her laugh. Perhaps it was just that I wasn't one of them—not Bermuda, not the family. Or because I talked about books so much, for all she seemed to do was stay in her rooms—another guest house, used to be the stablemaster's quarters—and read and read. Jane Austen for the second time, all of it, she who might've been Elizabeth Bennett herself, or Emma Wood- house, though not so willful. Party to the same invitations, same social order, same intrigues. I'd never really thought of them as guidebooks before.

Megs loved to talk about the moral ironies of that other age. She would come down to the beach with the rest of us, but always in a kind of sarong, because of the scars. (She swam in the Sound by herself late at night, the family said.) We'd sit in the shade of a coral arch and gab. Not gossip, not anything terribly personal—which was fine with me, as deep in the closet as I could get, Houdini chained in a trunk underwater but with no incentive to escape. No, books were the safest thing by far; except of course they lead in the end to matters philosophical.

The sun was nearly down, and everyone else had gone up to change. We'd reached a sort of companionable silence, Megs and I, as if all talk were taking a vespers break for the gold and lilac lightshow in the West. But then out of nowhere she spoke with a slow-burning passion: "Sometimes I wish I were anywhere else but here."

It took me a moment to parse it, unsuccessfully. "Here?" I echoed. "You mean the beach?"

"Oh, I don't know." She was scoffing at herself already, the moment's glimpse into her heart about to be over. "Ber- muda, I guess. These stodgy old colonels. The wives as brittle as teacups. Full of these hairline cracks."

"But where would you go instead?" I asked. She'd been everywhere else with Croesus, hadn't she?—everywhere else that was suitable for the princess class. And hadn't she left all

that behind to come back here like a lost Miranda to Pros-
pero's island? Too fragile for the world out there.

She laughed. "You know, my family used to be pirates.
Generations of them. Buccaneers—what's a buccaneer, exactly? Maybe I should go into the family business."

And the moment passed, before I could even form the
question, ask what it was that had trapped her so. The cancer?
But the only time she ever made mention of the gutting of
her insides was to toss it off lightly. "That was before they
took out all my ulcers," she said one day. "So now I never
worry, because I have nothing to worry with." With a quarter
smile that belied it all, even as she declared it. I was rendered
mute in the face of such crossed signals, rather like Mr.
Knightly himself.

It was the last full day of our two-week Easter break, with
nothing planned but a final scorch on the beach, to send us
home just a shade short of mahogany. We were all at the
breakfast table on the Harrington terrace, scarfing down
Grandmother's waffles swimming in Lyle's Golden Syrup. All
except Megs, who ate off a tray in her own quarters, at least
in the morning.

"It takes me an age to get going in the morning," she told
me once with characteristic breeziness. "Noon is about my
speed."

So imagine our collective shock when she appeared on
the terrace at nine A.M., and dressed to the nines besides.
Chanel suit, Ferragamo heels, and even a broad-brimmed linen
hat—she who usually stuck to sarongs and a cocktail shift for
the evening; never any jewelry at all, not even earrings—
sporting a diamond tennis bracelet and a black pearl choker
with earrings to match. Even Grandmother looked suitably
nonplussed.

"Megs," coaxed the teacher's wife, "come have a waffle."

Megs shook her head, smiling all the while in my direction. "But this one's going with me," she announced, crook-

ing a finger to beckon to me. "Can you bear to put on a tie?" I jumped up, prepared to put on three if necessary. "Meet me out by the garage," she said, "and I'll go see to lunch."

She drove an old wood-chassis Morgan—got it on her sixteenth birthday—its body mottled with rust and corrosion under its original racing green. The tattered top was down, Megs at the wheel. As I climbed in the other side, I saw in the space behind the bucket seats . . . the picnic hamper from the dairy auction, surfaced from a childhood cave of dreams. Not the very same, of course, but like enough that I told her the story, 157 and all. She responded with a sympathetic cluck and then a burst of laughter as the wind whipped through the car.

"Well, it's time you had a proper picnic, then."

We turned up the hill that looked out on Hamilton Harbor, the hill that held the manors of the old-line rich, the colonels and their teacups, pirates long expunged from the family tree. I thought, we must be going to a brunch or something, but then why the picnic finery? Megs turned in at a pair of cedar gates, with the drive parked up on either side with cars. At the crest of the rise she maneuvered the Morgan through the hedges and parked on the lawn. A trifle brazen, even for a princess.

As we got out, nearly trampling a bed of prize begonias, she murmured behind her hand: "Mother wouldn't come with me. They used to play bridge together. Every Friday, for decades."

Then she led the way round the side of the house, the opposite way from the front door. More hedges, and an overgrown arbor out of Edward Gorey (or Edward Lear), and we came out onto the sloping lawn in front, which proved to be chockablock with things—upholstered chairs, an elephant's foot umbrella stand, a rococo mirror leaning against a white-flowered tree, end tables and Tiffany lamps, armoires and steamer trunks—a total hodgepodge of life among the carriage trade.

Nailed to a column on the white veranda was a sign that pulled no punches: AUCTION BEGINS PROMPTLY AT ONE P.M. NO BIDDING WITHOUT A NUMBERED PADDLE.

So I wasn't a step behind anymore, except for trying to keep up with Megs, who drifted from piece to piece distractedly, running her fingers along the grain. When I caught up with her, she was standing next to a card table with a faded green baize inset. We whispered at the same moment: "The bridge table."

Then we made our way up the wide teak steps to the veranda—fifty more lots of bibelots, kitschy Dresden milkmaids, Waterford vases, that sort of thing. Megs cast a brief glance from thing to thing, then said as we passed inside: "This is what it all comes down to, you know. For all of them."

Of course she recognized several of the browsers, and they her. But there was a certain downcast look they shared, not quite catching one another's eyes—as if they'd been caught with their pants down, or their manners anyway. In the parlor above the fireplace was a portrait just like Megs's, a girl whose cheeks were flushed with running or riding or a morning's sail. I blurted out, unthinkingly: "How old was she?"

"When she died? Just turned eighty. Never sick a day in her life, till last year." She shook her head. "The end was torture."

And then we trailed up the circular stairs to the bedrooms. Stacks of old embroidered sheets, and table runners and doilies by the gross. In the master bedroom, with the balcony view of the harbor, silver brushes and beaded bags, onyx compacts, tortoise combs, each with a numbered tag. And medical gear besides: a walker, a nest of canes, a hospital bed. "Pathetic, isn't it," Megs declared, and we walked out onto the balcony. Gazing down at the yachted harbor, she began to recite, so softly I could hardly hear:

> She dwells with Beauty—Beauty that must die;
>   And Joy, whose hand is ever at his lips
> Bidding adieu . . .
> Aye, in the very temple of Delight
>   Veiled Melancholy has her sov'reign shrine. . . .

Keats, I promptly recognized. The "Ode on Melancholy," though I'd never much given it any thought since college, and certainly couldn't figure why she recalled it now. I would've guessed we'd come to the perfect place for

> . . . on the pedestal these words appear:
> "My name is Ozymandias, king of kings:
> Look on my works, ye Mighty, and despair!"
> Nothing beside remains.

Except this auction would be the woman's version—Ozymandia, queen of queens.

But the poetry lesson was over. We hastened back downstairs and out the door, as if Megs had been holding her breath the whole time we'd been inside. "It's quarter to twelve," she said. "We'd better go fetch the hamper."

As we came around to the side again, we could see that a safe had been brought out under the trees, the cast-iron kind with a double combination dial, the one that used to advertise how it survived the Chicago fire, or was it Hiroshima? A uniformed guard stood on either side.

"The jewelry," Megs remarked sardonically, and we headed back to the car to retrieve the picnic. She let me carry it, the wicker nicely creaking against my thigh, and led the way down a garden alley that ran below the house. I saw where we were bound for now: a white gazebo on the point of the bluff, not visible from the house. It could've used a paint job, and the ceiling corners were caked with mud, swallows' nests. But the wrought-iron table and chairs were sturdy, and the first thing out of the hamper was an embroidered linen tablecloth, with napkins to match.

Then the heavy silver and the Wedgewood china—we were worlds away from a Glennie's picnic; thirty-five hundred milk stoppers would've barely covered a spoon in Megs's kit. We opened a bottle of Mumm's and clinked a toast, though Megs took only the barest sip, on account of her missing stomach. But I was happy to drink the rest, toasting the yachts below and the anxious swallows who flew in and out above our heads. I don't even recall what we ate, only the sensory overload of the service, the sterling tines against my tongue.

"So what should we bid on?" I asked. "The bridge table?"

Megs frowned in distaste. "Nothing at all. I don't want any more *things,* do you?"

Oh, I did, but I lied. Nicely parroting back her breeziest air: "You're right. It's all just baggage, isn't it?"

"Exactly. Besides, haven't you learned your lesson yet? There are never enough milk stoppers."

We sat silent a while in the shady pavillion. Then—I must've had half the bottle by that point—I began to wax sentimental. "I promise to write when I get home," I declared with vinous fervor. "Maybe we can start on the Brontës together. And I'll be back, of course. We'll see each other again."

She paused for what felt like minutes, though the smile— her ineffable smile, as always—never wavered. "No, we won't," she retorted at last. "You have all your other things to write. And anyway, *you*'ve got to go be a buccaneer. *Somebody* has to." It was all very playful, of course; but even I, with my head full of bubbles, knew we were saying goodbye. Without rancor, without even melancholy. It was just what it was.

She didn't go with the rest of us to the airport in the morning, but she made an appearance as we packed our gear into Grandmother's Rover, saronged again but well before noon. She went around the half-circle of us and pecked both our cheeks in the French manner. I was the last and got no different kisses from the others. But she held my shoulders a moment longer and met my eyes.

"Maybe someday," she smiled, "you'll write an ode for me."

And that, as they say, was the long and the short of it. The end of Megs and me, of Bermuda and me, and the closest I ever came to an Empress in the flesh. That last spring term at Sutton Hill was as dingy as ever, cruel and stupid bureaucrats making all their administrative fuss, picking at nits, as they sent their overprivileged charges out into the world. Meanwhile the entire lot of us young Turk drudges quit *en masse,* dispersing to the four winds. I kept up for a while with my friend who was Megs's nephew, but then he and his wife split up, and he married the high school babysitter who'd gone along on our mid-ocean Easter jaunt. I had no connection left to Grandmother's pirate kingdom, hadn't even taken down the address.

And what was I supposed to send a letter about? My crazy years at Canton Academy, struggling out of the closet like a chrysalis? When Megs would cross my mind, I'd think: she's probably gone by now. I'd never quite believed the cancer while I was there, but afterward I put it all together—the fateful things she always said—and couldn't believe otherwise.

I remained in the Keatsian family business for another half-decade, but I never did write Megs's ode. Not good enough to, among other things, and not exactly gasping like Keats and coughing up blood. As for Megs's fond prediction that I would go into the buccaneer trade, surely I'd have disappointed her there as well. As fate would have it, I've written her story instead; and as fate would have it double, I've written it moored in the coral lagoon in Bora Bora, and now under sail to Moorea. Buccaneer country, no doubt about it, but I haven't a cutlass and don't wear a headrag, not even a gold hoop earring. Back home I live in a pirate's shark pit, but these are pirates in Armani suits, no coral harbor to anchor in, no sea breeze to muss their hair.

But I'd like to be able to tell her I finally got her lesson on *things*. It took me a couple of decades, and too much time among the gross excesses of people with a great deal more loot than consciousness. And it isn't that I don't like presents, both the giving and the getting, especially at Christmas—still silently counting how many. But things that are anvils tied to the ankles while a body is trying to swim—enough of those. I don't need any more evidence that riches end up in bank vaults.

And I'd like her to know how free she seemed on that long-ago Easter break—despite the gutting of her insides, and an air of otherworldly strangeness and isolation that must have left her feeling quite alone. And yet the glimmer in her eyes when she was quiet affirmed, it seemed, a deep core of liberation somewhere in her heart, like a white bird soaring. Maybe I'm not so free as that, but I have to say I'm as rid of chattels as I can be, here in the sailing lanes of an earthly paradise. Nothing in vaults. Even if it's an illusion, experience alone feels like the one thing slightly ahead of mortal, sometimes a bare footfall ahead. The rest is baggage. And Megs was the one who taught me that.

In this respect, especially, Winston's my ace in the hole. One thing's sure, there won't be a yard sale after I'm gone. I like giving stuff away. We haven't quite reached the stage where if you tell me something's pretty—picking it up off an end table—it's yours, and over your protests I will be wrapping it in tissue and tucking it into a bag. Not quite yet; but the notion is appealing, placing all my things like orphans, finding them good homes.

And yet, perversely, I can't imagine leaving behind my Dorothea Lange and my Ansel Adams, or the pebble on my desk from Delphi, fetched from the icy bed of the Kastalian Spring. Or even my gray Italian cardigan lined with satin — so threadbare, so worn in, it makes me look as seedy and eccentric as any old Boston Brahmin coupon-clipper. These things aren't just mine, these things are indistinguishable from me.

Well, we'll see how far I get with my dispersal of the goods, and otherwise Winston will keep what constitutes a home, not including some few pieces to be carted off to my brother and sister-in-law. Intact enough, my furnishings, that they won't be picked over by estate-sale sluts. Not that Mrs. Hamilton Harbor could have cared in her last draconian year, mostly confined to her bedroom and hospital gear at the end. The last of the line, no children, with maybe a scant third cousin who could summon neither a sigh of regret nor a grasping lust for all that post-Victorian clutter. Who needs eighty doilies? Let them go to the highest bidder, with the ghosts and carriage-trade etiquette in the bargain.

Inexorably, somehow, the moral of that story transports me into the thick of another parable, twenty years after Bermuda and seven years into AIDS. The barony in question was on the Gold Coast of Long Island, so-called by the robber millionaires themselves as they built their Norman chateaux and Tudor manors, their Grand Trianons and Scottish castles. A thousand of them, constructed in the heady years between the century's turn and the Crash, once lined Long Island Sound. Thirty years of Gatsby-itis, including the model for the Old Sport's place itself, Fitzgerald's dream vision of *ultima Thule*.

And when the fuck-you money disappeared, the houses became just so many white elephants, requiring staffs of sixty or eighty and sit-down dinners for half a hundred. Abandoned to taxes, boarded up and vandalized, the Tiffany cathedral ceilings shattered, the stone-carved balustrades carted off piecemeal to a later suburban hell, the marble gods and goddesses at the center of the mazes rendered headless, an age of property stripped of gilt like the statue of *The Happy Prince* in Oscar Wilde.

Some stand in ruins still, recorded in all their rotting splendor by Monica Randall in *The Mansions of Long Island's Gold Coast*.[4] Of that thousand in their prime, perhaps a few dozen are left, inhabited by think tanks and cloistered religious orders and the random secret diplomatic corps. In the eighties Randall identified only eight still held in private hands. And one of these, on a marsh-rimmed island just off Glen Cove, is the subject of our sermon here—an AIDS sermon, as it happens, though we'll come to that twist presently. As they say in the picture business, first we have to fill in the backstory.

Originally constructed for a Midas banker of the Morgan class, a titan who struck a deal with the City of New York to construct the Holland Tunnel and keep the excavated stone. Which was barged in giant slabs worthy of the Pyramids to this thirty-acre island forty minutes from Manhattan. (Forty minutes today; the weekend guests then would arrive more languidly by water.) From the iron-gray bedrock they built a house of fifty-five rooms, walls three feet thick, with wings extending from an earldom of public salons, embracing two acres of lawn that front the Sound, shaded by oaks and sycamores. From the dock one proceeded across the lawn, trailed by bearers with steamer trunks to a fountained formal entrance.

The landscape architect was Olmsted, late of Central Park, who laid out the thirty acres with an eye to what effect they'd make a quarter century later. The vast English garden lay on the inland side of the house, with a triple allée of hedges and borders and blossoming trees. Including the largest weeping beech on Long Island—or was it North America?—with a

---

4. New York: Rizzoli International Publications, 1979; revised, 1987.

suite of outdoor furniture in the shady tent of branches reaching to the ground. Ideal for a summer *tête-à-tête* out of Edith Wharton. Stables and kennels and greenhouses and barns and a folly, all manner of cutting gardens and vegetables, all out of sight of the house.

Midas and Missus entertained in twenties ducal style, five-day weekends, all that. They even kept their assets through the thirties, when everyone else's bankers were leaping out of windows and selling apples on street corners. Midas died in the seventies, fat and gouty, leaving the place to his wife— who promptly had a stroke or two .and ended in a nursing home eating off paper plates. Her own three golden children had long since ceased to speak to Ma and Pa, and as for inheritance wanted no part of a white elephant. Either sell it whole or tear it down and subdivide. For some years there was a standoff, as the stone edifice in the salt marsh grew emptier and emptier. When a prospective buyer decided to offer a bid, he'd only seen the place from a helicopter, and understood there were certain conditions to the sale.

He visited the shriveling widow in her tiny private cell at the Golden Crest convalescent facility, from which no one escaped alive. She was sipping her Postum from a styrofoam cup, she who'd had a dozen different china patterns in the old days, service for a hundred right down to the fingerbowls. A photograph of the mansion—which only she called by its proper name, *East Wind*—was perched on the tray table between the Kleenex and the bedpan. Though more than slightly balmy, speaking garbled words out of the side of her mouth, she told him the house needed lots of work. But she wanted it saved so badly that she'd bargain-basement the price.

"But it's not *East Wind* itself that matters now," she said, and fixed him with rheumy eye and the clutch of a palsied hand. "Mr. Hall, say you'll take care of my dogs till they die, and *East Wind* is yours."

More than the china and the Gobelin upholstery and

the Coromandel screens, she missed her brood of Labradors. When Arthur Hall said yes, he didn't know the black Lab population was forty-five; but he saw a shiver of near ecstatic relief transform the old lady's face, the very last thing finally settled.

"May you be as happy as we were there," she managed to choke through tears. Having outlived happiness for what must have seemed like a century. And no, the head nurse curtly informed Arthur on his way out, they didn't allow their ladies to be visited by dogs.

So. The very same cautionary tale as Bermuda, right down to the fingerbowls and the bedpan. Not as if one really needed to hear it again. There is of course the additional twist of Mrs. Midas's final throes, something I was spared at the Hamilton Harbor rummage sale. And of course the dogs themselves—the old ones gone within a year, the young ones penned in their kennel runs, or walked in packs along the shore, baying in unison like a hunt—for close to a decade. What had *they* outlived exactly, assuming the kibble and scraps were up to par?

Or is that just more of the simpering bathos of Western culture, that envies a dog for needing no possessions and, in the next breath, scathes the human dispossessed for causing all their own misery? It surely needs no pointing out that everyone here—from Harrington Sound to *East Wind,* indeed all the way to Cook's Bay in Moorea—has more than enough of everything. Mountains more.

But that only makes the cautionary tale more pertinent to the global tidal wave of poverty and genocide, economic slavery and genital mutilation. For the victims—for virtually everyone, that is—the proper response to all of this is Shelley's gloating sneer:

> My name is Ozymandias, king of kings:
> Look on my works, ye Mighty, and . . .

. . . have a good laugh. The problems of doilies and knuckle-sized emeralds, even of cardigan sweaters, are fodder for a cosmic joke.

And yet the fall of the high and mighty satisfies some fundamental human need—as Sophocles and Shakespeare knew, masters of the art of *Schadenfreude*. We have to believe the rich will get theirs, their things picked over by jackals and buzzards, or we could scarcely bear the pitiful cache of milk stoppers that constitutes the sum of our earthly goods. Because we resist believing that riches are next to godliness, despite the huckstering of the God squad, who could easily find some Jesus-y use for the eighty doilies, but who much prefer negotiable securities—the ticket of priestly commerce that ensures a rich man's passage through the needle's eye, and all his camels besides.

We resist it, all right, even though the evidence is so much on the other side—the trappings of their baronies, the ceaseless banqueting, the platinum credit cards, and themselves as likely as not to reach their eighties and nineties still possessed of everything. Republican thieves especially (talk about pirates), and shahs and caliphs and despots, in the banking trade or otherwise. No, we have to believe they'll die alone, unmourned, in agony, their useless diamonds glittering through their seizures, splashed with the blood they cannot keep from coughing up. We need their bad deaths writ very large, or how could we ever let go ourselves?

But back to *East Wind* and the sermon in its stones. It was my friend Craig, freelance pauper and journalist, who stumbled onto it. At his AIDS support group meeting in a West Village vestry hall, he struck up a friendship with one James Merion—the two of them having established that they had about the same number of immune cells left (basically none) and a more or less equal body count of KS lesions and dead friends. Thus equally far along the road, they sat to a cappuccino. Craig was hating New York in the summer, and was too penniless for a stint in the Pines.

"Well," offered James, "then you should come out to Glen Cove. We have a big house there."

To put it mildly. As soon as Craig saw the scope of Midas's gold he turned into the man who came to dinner, spending nearly every four-day weekend at *East Wind,* and usefully besides. For the owner, Arthur Hall, supported his and James's life in the castle harbor by means of weekly business jaunts to London, Rome, and the Persian Gulf, where he was a major buccaneer in the oil trade. And he genuinely worried over leaving his lover alone, even in a mansion crawling with help, no matter if James protested he was happy just tending the garden—that is, overseeing an outdoor staff of eight and a resident botanist besides. Craig had therefore found his situation, as a semi-permanent AIDS buddy.

Through the whole of 1986 Craig waxed delirious about *East Wind,* playing it for all it was worth like a lifesize game of *Clue*—Miss Scarlet in the conservatory with the lead pipe. I was happy for him, unambiguously so, knowing how his lust for a taste of baronial life had never been quite assuaged. That is, he'd never had his Bermuda. Regrettably, though, his weekly reports from the island coincided with Roger's last six months. I was in a frenzy of throwing out books whenever I wasn't occupied pumping Roger with IV meds or with the endless round of doctors' appointments—unless we were actually doing time in solitary on the tenth floor at UCLA. *Vanity of vanities . . . all is vanity* was more or less my take on the bulletins from the Gold Coast.

"You and Roger just have to come out here!" Craig would wax enthusiastic without thinking. Roger was all but blind by that point, and stricken by the loss of his own hillside patch of garden. We needed thirty acres like a hole in the head. Sardonically, in my own pre-mourning desperation, I privately disdained the pleasures of *East Wind,* doubting they would make a day of difference to the speed of all our dying.

I didn't get there myself till the following summer, nine

months after burying Roger and only a little less raving mad and death-haunted, not exactly ready to be a houseguest. Like Heathcliff invited for a tennis weekend. But *East Wind* proved to be every bit as boggling as Craig had painted it—library out of Conan Doyle, music room hung with tapestries of the Muses, suites of silken bedchambers. One of the garden crew's main jobs when the owners were in residence was splitting and stocking wood for the thirty-two fireplaces, including the Lilliputian one in my bath. All set to be lit in case of a June chill.

As the synergy of AIDS would have it, I liked James Merion right away, though somehow Craig had never said how purple he was, with lesions rampant. And so bone-thin you could practically see right through him to the candlelight behind him on the sideboard. "I hope they told you," he drawled, "that I look like E.T.'s brother."

He was thoroughly unpretentious, a pianist with impeccable credentials, but he'd fallen away from his music since turning purple, at least when it came to giving recitals. He mostly delighted in conducting tours of the gardens and the quarter mile of shoreline by golf cart, lacking the strength to walk his acreage now. Appearing to know the botanical minutiae of every leaf and sprout.

But at meals in the Roman-painted dining room, the discussion was every bit as maddened over AIDS and the straights' indifference as it was anywhere gay men gathered. Obsessively following up on the latest treatments and pipe-dream rumors. *East Wind* turned out to be a safehouse, boiling over with last-ditch schemes and anarchic plots, like an ACT UP meeting in Versailles. Or we'd assemble together in the walnut-paneled parlor to hear James's latest blood counts— never good—and help him negotiate a course like so many outlaw biochemists, even as a formal tea was being laid out by the under-butler.

AIDS was the canker in the rose of *East Wind*, but after

Bermuda the juxtaposition of sybaritic and mortal made a kind of cockeyed sense. And the walks we took at night, Craig and I—Arthur, too, if he was in from London, living as he did in a state of permanent jet lag—were the closest talks I ever had about dying. With the salt breeze off the marshes and the flash of herons rising into the moonlight, we made a certain provisional peace with the nightmare that would never leave us now. More death talk than I ever had with Roger, with whom I'd groped to stay alive with a murderous single-mindedness, our fingers pulped to bloody stumps from clawing up the mountain.

James was dying before our eyes, but Craig and I still had a ways to go. So what was left? And how would we bear it? And how bear the banalities of everyone's well-meaningness, especially the seronegatives'?

I went out there again in October, an overnight with Craig on our way to Tuscany. James was weaker than ever, a half-sleep taking up the heart of his days at *East Wind*. And yet still able to draw the strength for the golf-cart circuit of the gardens, the trees aching with color in the blue-gold light of autumn, roses still at their peak, and flights of Canada geese stopping over in the marshes as they headed south. Even then James was engaged in a massive garden project, the laying out and planting of the longest perennial border in Long Island—or was it North America? I didn't expect that James would see it through, though he had his gardeners bustling like the Queen's in *Alice*. I also didn't think I would be seeing James again.

And didn't. He died on a bright cold day in February, Valentine's Day in fact, in Arthur's arms, Arthur's children and James's Virginia family grouped about the bed in a sad half-circle. Arthur propped him up so he could see to the Sound at sunset, the great lawn blanketed in snow, and then it was over.

It was decided to wait till the roses bloomed again for the memorial service, and I surely thought it would mark the end of our days on the Gold Coast. I couldn't imagine Arthur keeping the place alone, so inextricably linked as it was with James and suffused with the echoes of Liszt and Chopin. And besides, Arthur was having to spend more time in the sheik-doms of Arabia.

I hadn't counted on his—what? Generosity is hardly the word. On the life-force decision to let Craig come and go the same as ever, the skeleton staff instructed to keep the house ready and stocked for the random sojourns of my penniless friend.

And thus began a different age, for *East Wind* and for us. I came back later that winter and again in the first dogwood flush of spring. The east wind was indeed a biting presence then, whipping in off the water, giving our walks a Wuthering edge. But the wind was no match for those three-foot walls of stone and the roaring fires we sat by, room after room. It wasn't as if we felt we owned it in any real way, or that we harbored a secret fantasy that here at least we were safe from the Valley of the Shadow; or that we'd be doing this season after season, no end in sight. No—*East Wind* was just for now, but now was all we had.

And the talk of dying came to be a way of talking out our lives, how we'd loved and whom we'd failed, and what was the legacy of this pointless suffering we had witnessed and en-dured. I'd met Craig, after all, the very same night I met Roger, and nobody else could quite replace so much history shared. We knew we were the last of *our* kind, come of age in the seventies. The very last queers of a certain caste of mind— formed in the crucible of revolution, yet trailing in our wake the gaudy streamers of Mardi Gras, a certain carnal swagger, and the last grace notes of Judy and the Ridiculous Theatre Company. Not all of it lost once we were gone, but the loss of what it all meant.

East Wind was our last refuge before the millennial rum-mage sale, a philosophical stroll through marbled halls, still prone to the camp imagining that we were a couple of dukes

ourselves. In June the memorial service played itself out among
the roses, accompanied by tapes of James at the piano. I had
written a proper elegy for James, but in the end was too sick—
a danger flag in my lungs—to fly back and deliver it myself. I
went back later that summer when Arthur was in residence
alone, grieving after his fashion—which was invisible under
his so unflappable charm, with its overlay of discretion and still
waters. But *East Wind* wasn't the same, and he knew it, and
Craig and I couldn't make it the same.

Finally not even for ourselves. By the last days of that summer I'd become involved with Stephen, and I brought him
with me when we were invited out to *East Wind* for Thanksgiving. Arthur's daughter was using the occasion to announce
her engagement, and she filled the house with friends and
oversaw a banquet—as in the old days, almost, or the old old
days of the Midases. Craig had his regular room, and I had
mine; but the presence of so many others, Stephen especially,
left Craig and me feeling a bit estranged.

I remember sitting with Stephen in the music room, reading Coleridge to him, "Frost at Midnight." Craig poked his
head in, saw right away the lay of the land, and turned to
go—over our protests, especially Stevie's, who'd had his fill of
Coleridge. But Craig just waved it off and headed upstairs for
a nap. My friend who would've gladly given up *East Wind* and
all its playing fields to have a lover to read to. He was fraying
around the edges now himself, slowing down like an unwound
clock—though in fact, of course, his AIDS clock had started
speeding up.

Still, we had a weekend to ourselves four months later,
over the blustering Ides of March. Walking our acreage yet
again. Though the island had not ceased to feel like a second
home, Craig admitted he was considering a move to Boston
where we'd all started from, it seemed a century ago. Nobody
traveled lighter than Craig, whose life's accumulation would
fit neatly in a rucksack. Besides, he said, he'd had it up to here

with New York, and the endless wait in waiting rooms. *East Wind* wasn't enough of a compensation anymore, especially being there alone.

Our swan song came in the middle of June, over Gay Pride Weekend. Arthur was in from Saudi, and the roses were at full blast. "I'll still be able to get down here whenever I want," Craig assured me as we lounged on the steps of the Moorish folly, shirtless and sunning in the glare off the Sound. But we both knew scheduling a visit together would be geometrically more complicated. Stevie was napping away in a hammock under the sycamores, seeming to understand instinctively that Craig and I needed to be alone to say goodbye. Not to each other yet—that was still more than a year away— but to all of this. To the dreamscape in all its midsummer effusion, and the fall of titans that had left *East Wind* to us for a time, a couple of boho queers.

And the rest is so predictable, it hardly bears repeating. For by the time the clock had wound itself so tight as to burst its springs, what had been unendurable tragedy for so long had now begun to feel most cruelly banal. Stevie and Craig were both beginning the final year, the exhausting mechanics of staying half alive. Stevie was finally taken out in September 1990, followed by Craig just after New Year's. No sunset over the great lawn, no herons in the marsh, no crackling fire by the bathtub. Just more tubes and choking oxygen feeds and the creeping up of the morphine drip.

I never heard from Arthur again, but understood he'd acquitted himself with honor throughout, holding off the final disposition of *East Wind* till its last sentinel was gone. I could take care of myself, he knew that. And when, some months later, a friend called excitedly to tell me the place was up for sale—an aerial view of the Midas kingdom in all the toniest realty listings—I hardly reacted at all. The cautionary tale in which you-can't-take-it-with-you was so engrained in me that I couldn't quite comprehend how the moral of it had changed.

For me anyway. Something to do with the final overcoming of that 157. Or passing the windows at Hammacher Schlemmer and barely glancing at the picnic hamper laid out in its finery. I see the difference now between mere baggage and what the heart possesses. Not that the latter is any less stolen goods—the brimming of love and the joy of a comrade—requiring every bit of a pirate's brazen stealth. And no less snatched in the end by the icy clutch of Death than all the baronies and all their rummage.

But the heart transformed in the process, no longer just a thing that ticks and no longer simply mortal, though half in shadow already. There's a cautionary tale in there as well, perhaps, involving a soul-deep self-delusion—but not worth the caution anyway. Something lasts, firm as the pen in my hand. Jackals and buzzards cannot get at it. Its price doesn't translate into dollars. Saved as it is in the spending, till nothing's left in the vault. Invisible in the blinding shine of the setting sun, weightless as a mid-ocean breeze. To have greatly loved is to sail without ballast—with neither chart nor cargo, not bound for the least of kingdoms. Nothing remains, except this being free.

SOME
AFTERTHOUGHTS

THE ESSAYS GATHERED here were written over the course of a year and a half, between August of 1992 and New Year's Eve, 1993. They appear in the order of composition—not so much because they were conceived as a thematic sequence as that I feared my illness would stop the project in mid-stride. A romantic presumption, having as its source *The Last Tycoon,* Fitzgerald's unfinished novel—cut short by a coronary in a house about six blocks from me. Leaving behind a mere scatter of notes as to what would have followed, and ending with his famous dictum, all in caps: ACTION IS CHARACTER. Or Dickens, who slumped at his half-acre desk before he could finish *The Mystery of Edwin Drood,* leaving the identity of the murderer eternally in doubt.

But of course those books were published anyway, filled out with notes and literary guesswork, and especially poignant to their readers by the very fact of their incompleteness. I was under no illusion that my own work-in-progress would qualify for the Dickens/Fitzgerald treatment. I figured I had to get more than halfway through to make it worth publication by

fragment. And it wasn't just lofty thoughts about the pantheon
of the unfinished Greats that proved such a goad to "Work,
for the night is coming," as the Protestant hymnal has it. No,
it had more to do with the generation of the incomplete to
which AIDS had consigned me—a legion of my fellow writers
from Robert Ferro to Allen Barnett, Bo Huston to Vito
Russo, all of them snatched mid-sentence.

Working under the gun, in other words, two years now
since being diagnosed with full-blown AIDS. Leashed to three
separate IV drugs and a small mountain of oral medication. I
don't offer this, not consciously, to seek the reader's sympathy
or forbearance. But it does explain why I never had the slightest idea what the next essay would be till I finished the one
before. Beginning each with a blank slate, and perhaps a stray
anecdote or two waiting in the wings. As much as possible,
then, letting the text itself take me where it went till I more
or less stumbled on a theme.

In one sense I am being disingenuous, of course, since the
subtext first to last—and not so very sub at all—serves as a
kind of picaresque chronology of the progression of disease
and treatment. It had been suggested to me before I began this
work that I might just keep a diary of AIDS, one man's eye-
witness report from the battlefront. But I felt as if I'd been
doing nothing but that for years and years and didn't have the
stomach for *World War III, Part V*. Besides, others had covered
that waterfront all along. From Emmanuel Dreuilhe to Paul
Reed and George Whitmore, urgent personal witness that
stood on the shelves with the history of the plague—Randy
Shilts's definitive *And the Band Played On*—and the work of
its various analysts, notably Douglas Crimp and Susan Sontag,
and John Preston's compendium of *Personal Dispatches: Writers
Confront AIDS*.

What I wanted to do instead was look at the vectors of
my life, the people and places and politics that had stuck with
me, resonant still despite the deluge of the last twelve years of

calamity. How had it changed the way I looked at things? Had anything survived intact? And did anything mean the same anymore? I had never started a book with so little strategy aforethought, or worked so much from instinct.

And everything *had* changed. Not surprisingly, my rabid contempt for official religions, the Orwellian lies and the Kapos, had only deepened over time. The entropy inherent in what was still quaintly called the civilized world continued geometrically toward utter disintegration. For mine was a classic *fin-de-siècle* gloom, Henry Adams without the education, convinced the world was just about over. Which put me in bed with the real wackos—the millennial Christian cults and the Rapturists—the difference being that the end of *my* civilization was as much their fault as the ozone hole or the plummet toward universal illiteracy or the opening of the hundred millionth McDonald's.

My ranting therefore didn't surprise me a bit. What took me more than slightly aback was discovering just how much certain people and incidents and feelings had only grown more precious over time. Had mattered more and changed me more than I'd ever quite acknowledged. Sources of affirmation that reflected, as in a mirror, the self I hoped to be—and incidentally serving to light the way of the checkered heart.

Of course, nothing stands still either. I would have to issue a daily bulletin to keep up with the burgeoning scandal of the pedophile priests, even as the Polish Pope has publicly tried to shift the blame to the anarchy of permissiveness. Society's to blame. Or, as one of the mealy Neo-Con apologists for the Church has written, we end up with the priests we deserve. It's our own damned fault. How's *that* for spin control? Mark Twain would've loved the gobbledygook in all of this: call it the spiritual equivalent of the Twinkie defense.

Fortuitously, by way of counterforce, there are certain heartening updates to report since the writing of these pieces. The Episcopal Bishop who came for tea last winter, for

instance, took Winston's advice and came out to the House of
Bishops. In his own way, of course: quietly sending an epistle
to his colleagues just before the general meeting of the House,
this year in Panama. In part he wrote:

> I have promised myself that I will not remain silent,
> invisible, unknown. After all is said and done, the
> choice for me is not whether or not I am a gay man,
> but whether or not I am honest about who I am with
> myself and others. It is a choice to take down the wall
> of silence I have built around an important and vital
> part of my life, to end the separation and isolation I
> have imposed on myself all these years.[1]

Thus did Bishop Otis Charles—I can name him now for
real, unlike so many of his fellow divines in "My Priests,"
identified pseudonymously so as not to incur an Inquisition—
become the first Bishop of any mainline denomination to dis-
close publicly the truth of his sexual orientation. An important
moment in gay and lesbian history, and a ringing challenge to
the status quo of invisibility. The reception to his coming out
can be imagined. In Panama several Bishops embraced him for
his courage, while others averted their faces and would not
meet his eyes.

Still, a beginning. Personally, we retain our precarious balance on Kings Road. It's a year now since Victor—fellow
traveler and soulmate—managed to save Puck's life when it
was hanging by a thread. Winston and I were in Big Sur just
after the turn of the year, dozing by the fire with a pummeling
rain on the roof, the glorious deep of winter. Back in Los
Angeles, Puck went out in the garden in the thick of the

---

1. From a news release by the *Episcopal News Service,* quoted in an interview
with Jeffrey Penn, Assistant News Director.

storm, nothing unusual in that, but Victor realized some minutes later that he hadn't come back in. He discovered Puck lying beneath the tree ferns at the top of the garden. He coaxed the dog inside, only to have Puck collapse on the kitchen floor, near comatose. A quick call to the Westside Animal Hospital, where the receptionist said it sounded like "bloat," requiring immediate surgery. Victor and a friend carried Puck's deadweight eighty-five pounds to the car and raced across town. As the dog was whisked into the operating room, Victor was given to understand that he'd made it just in time. Ten minutes later and Puck would have been gone.

Bloat is a desperate and sudden condition, in which the bowel somehow twists and cuts off digestion, quickly becoming gangrenous, killing within an hour. I never quite got the details right, but Victor's call is indelibly etched in the fault zone of my brain. Puck was still in surgery, but they thought they'd got it in time. The hour's wait for the post-op call was unbearable, like waiting for test results in the AIDS ward— what fresh hell were we entering now? Winston took it harder than I. In terror and anguish he kept repeating we needed all four of us dogs intact—or how would we ever mount the constant struggle with the horrors of AIDS? I understood exactly what he meant: the human/canine magic circle somehow kept us safe, no breaks in the line permitted or we were lost.

Puck came through it fine. And next day Winston and I drove eight hours straight through the buffeting wind and rain so we could see him during the one-hour window of time allowed for "family visits." We found him still very groggy in his cage, a fifteen-inch incision in his belly, but managing a plucky wag when he recognized us. Twenty-four hours later he was fully alert and clamoring for release— *Get me out of this place!*—and dashed that we had to leave him for another night of observation.

In other words, an AIDS emergency with a happy ending for once, even if the virus wasn't directly implicated. Puck has

lived out his thirteenth year—in dog years a veritable Methu-
selah—without further incident. He is more than just a little
deaf now, can't roam the canyon on his own anymore. The
Kings Road doghouse has accommodated him with a fenced-
in yard and security gate. His perch is the same at the top of
the outside stairs. He keeps watch, his hearing loss having tri-
pled the decibel count of his warning bark. People who pass
the house, trudging uphill, cross the road to the other side so
as not to get him started.

My own bark has grown softer of late, but that's because
I've already scared off most of that class of intruders and tres-
passers who get too close. For all of that, my rage at my lost
country is undiminished, but I choose my shouting matches
carefully these days, husbanding my energy and adrenaline for
the war going on inside me. Meanwhile, the dying continues
unabated. Michael Callen gone three weeks ago—mid-song as
it were—after twelve years in the trenches. In yesterday's
Times an obit for my friend Dan Bailey, one of the founding
fathers of Gay Men's Health Crisis, the gentlest man imaginable, and there is no one I can call for details because all of
our mutual acquaintance is dead.

Three weeks, two dead—two more lost from the magic circle. Or, to put it another way, two more rocks flung at the vast
glass house of the world's complacency—falling short as usual.
But then the numbers of the disappeared are relative at best, and
buried in a thicket of lies they call statistics. Or, as Randall Jarrell
put it succinctly, counting the bodies of another war:

> We died on the wrong page of the almanac . . .
> When we died they said, "Our casualties were low."[2]

---

2. Randall Jarrell, *The Complete Poems* (New York: Farrar, Straus and Giroux,
1969), page 145.

As for my own losses, the pile of bodies is hardly countable anymore except in the heart—because the dead outnumber the living now. Personally, that is.

Which brings me to the subtitle of this book, in the interest of providing context. Just after the '93 March on Washington, I had a call from the *pukka sahib* of a prominent national weekly, asking if I would care to write a piece on the week's events. I said it was the very thing I was planning to do next, but demurred that I was probably looking at fifty pages and two months' work. Not news enough by then—not hot enough—for their purposes, I imagined. She quickly countered that time and length were not a problem. I should send it along once it was finished to my satisfaction. She assured me she was a great admirer of my work.

Flush from so much flattery, I nevertheless replied with a poke of irony. Maybe she hadn't heard, I told her, but her staff had already rejected two of the essays, "Gert" and "My Priests."

"Who did that?" she retorted, a bit defensive, clearly having been left out of the loop. "And why?"

"They said my work was too personal." Oh, she didn't like that at all, but then I hadn't the least idea who the editorial culprits were. And besides, this whole exchange had put me in a state of merry *bonhomie*. "It's all right, really," I assured her. "You have to understand that I spent twenty years being turned down because my work was considered 'too gay.' Which I came to regard as a compliment, and proof I was on the right track."

Now, due to the geometric growth of the literature of my people—not to mention the imprimatur of the National Book Award—I had presumably outlived any lingering curse at being so dismissed. Except now I'd become "too personal," which I couldn't help but feel was even better than a compliment. For I grew up in a culture in which the personal was *verboten,* especially in polite company—a company I've long since sold my stock in. So what looked like another rejection slip was as much a cause for celebration.

I don't know that she followed the logic there, being as her calls on hold were clamoring like hungry dogs. Ever gracious nevertheless, she urged me on and told me please to always keep them in mind.

But in fact the real dismissal has come from much closer to home. It's probably no surprise, but the gay and lesbian nation has lately spun off a particularly nasty subspecies of Neo-Con dissent. A sourpuss brand of critic who rejects the very notion of "gay." Their homosexuality, they say, is the least of their defining characteristics, rather like having brown eyes instead of blue. Thus they disdain gay pride and its carnival exuberance, and find our politics rude and out of bounds, especially the unseemly spread of the gay "subculture." For God's sake, can't we be more discreet? No wonder so many decent people hate us.

These are exclusively the views of conservative men, who are the first to admit they cannot speak for lesbians, since they don't know any. Of course they imply that AIDS is all our own subcultural fault, and just deserts for our libertine ways. But which of us is the stereotype here? The meek and proper clerks and choirboys, undercooked and undisclosed, assimilationist at all costs? *Don't ask, don't tell* so deeply engrained, they can sport it as a serial tattoo when the camps are ready.

No sense of the multifaceted community we have forged, or the systems we have put in place to care for our own, or the common vow we have made to stop the silence. They're welcome to their free speech, of course, and welcome to rub shoulders with the pundits and think-tankers of the right, as well as the church supper crowd of the Christian Reich. Time alone will tell whether resistance or collaboration is more in our best interests as a people. For the present, by all means let them be not gay, not gender-variant, not ghettoized, with nary a sequin to betray them. Prim and smug and Puritan by choice, far removed from any culture that smacks of sub.

But I give them fair warning that I for one am taking it all personally—too personally, in fact. Keeping a file of mealiness, of pandering to creeps, of accommodation with the enemy. I don't really have the choice to ignore it, because it's happening on my watch.

Printed in the United States
36812LVS00004B/169-174